PUBLIC HEALTH IN THE 21ST CENTURY

MIDWIFERY

GLOBAL PERSPECTIVES, PRACTICES AND CHALLENGES

PUBLIC HEALTH IN THE 21ST CENTURY

Additional books in this series can be found on Nova's website under the Series tab.

Additional e-books in this series can be found on Nova's website under the e-book tab.

PUBLIC HEALTH IN THE 21ST CENTURY

MIDWIFERY

GLOBAL PERSPECTIVES, PRACTICES AND CHALLENGES

GORDON DENNEL
EDITOR

nova publishers
New York

Additional color graphics may be available in the e-book version of this book.

Library of Congress Cataloging-in-Publication Data

Midwifery : global perspectives, practices and challenges / Editors: Gordon Dennel.
pages cm. -- (Public health in the 21st century)
Includes index.
ISBN: 978-1-63463-113-6 (hardcover)
1. Midwifery--Cross-cultural studies. I. Dennel, Gordon, editor.
RG950.M5249 2014
618.2--dc23 2014036533

Published by Nova Science Publishers, Inc. † New York

CONTENTS

PREFACE

The role of traditional midwives varies across cultures and at different times and even today these traditional practitioners attend the majority of deliveries in rural areas in developing countries. According to WHO, each year 45 million births occur at home without skilled health personnel. Skilled attendants assist in more than 99% of births in more developed countries, versus 62% in developing countries. In many rural and periurban communities, the perinatal care that traditional midwives offer is generally profoundly rooted in the local culture and collectively valuated as the result of hand-on experience. There is little doubt that traditional midwives play an important role when it comes to cultural competence, empathy and psychosocial support at birth with important benefits for the mother and the new-born baby. This book discusses global perspectives, practices and challenges involved in midwifery.

Chapter 1 – Public health programs in Latin America are encouraging the participation of traditional midwives in trainings programs on birth, delivery practices and risks reduction. Although the existing literature focuses on the health outcomes of training of traditional midwives, there is a paucity of research analyzing the perceptions and the acceptance of such training programs by traditional midwives.

What is the perception of midwives who have been trained vis-à-vis these training programs? Are these training programs an effective way to reduce the marginalization of traditional midwifery and to enhance stronger forms of collaboration between traditional medicinal systems and biomedicine? Or on the contrary are they a way to reinforce the dominance and dependence of traditional midwives towards biomedicine?

This chapter analyzes the way in which training programs in Ecuador and Mexico have transformed the role of traditional midwives and their perceptions of traditional midwifery identity and practices in their process of negotiation between traditional medicine and biomedicine.

Chapter 2 – Midwives are a key profession in the care of women during the childbearing process, and research results indicate that they can have a major effect upon their wellbeing and health as well as upon their attitude to future births and to their new born child. Women's need for *caring* in the childbearing process and the great importance of the *caring midwife* has been established by listening, through research, to women who have given birth. The detrimental effects of uncaring has also been demonstrated in the same way. What is caring then? What is uncaring? How can we recognize and avoid uncaring? More importantly, how can we teach caring and how can we help midwifery students to avoid being perceived as uncaring? Finally, how should midwifery education be organized in order to educate caring midwives? These are the basic questions the authors will try to answer in this discussion paper. The authors conclude that during revision of midwifery education programmes the focus should always be on how all the different aspects of the complicated project of educating a "good midwife" be included in the curriculum and that the importance of caring will not be left out.

Chapter 3 – Stress urinary incontinence (SUI), the complaint of involuntary loss of urine on effort, physical exertion, sneezing or coughing, is the most common type of urinary incontinence (UI) in pregnant women. The prevalence of SUI during pregnancy is reported by approximately 18.6% to 75% of all pregnant women. It is well known that SUI is related to reduced muscle strength, as well as the supportive and sphincteric function of the pelvic floor such as the pelvic floor muscles (PFM), connective tissue and fascia. Pregnancy is one of the main risk factors for the development of SUI. The physiological changes during pregnancy may lead to reduced strength of supportive and sphincteric function of the PFM.

SUI in pregnant women can be prevented and improved by intensive pelvic floor muscle exercise (PFME). Pregnant women who regularly and correctly perform PFME will have hypertrophy of muscle fibers with strengthening of the PFM and periurethral muscles leading to improvement of the sphincteric function efficiency and decreased urine leakage. However, some physicians suggest that intensive exercise by a therapist cannot be implemented into clinical practice. It is likely that the success of randomized controlled trials reported in the many research cannot be repeated in a `real clinical situation'.

Most pregnant women tend to consider SUI a common discomfort of pregnancy. Although they are often inconvenienced and troubled by SUI symptoms, they are reluctant to seek help from health professionals. The majority of pregnant women are not provided with information on SUI. During pregnancy, 55% percent of women receive some form of instruction in PFME. This means that not all pregnant women receive instruction about SUI and PFME during pregnancy. Moreover, the information is provided by a variety of health professionals and no single profession appears to undertake the responsibility of providing this service. Thus, it is suggested that midwives may not have a direct responsibility to provide this knowledge to pregnant women despite the fact that nurses or midwives are health professionals most closely involved with most pregnant women. Thus, to be effective in the prevention and treatment SUI during pregnancy by PFME, there is a need for the service to be reorganized to ensure that all pregnant women receive high-quality instruction during pregnancy. Midwives should assess the SUI symptoms in pregnant women and provide instruction about SUI and PFME during pregnancy in addition to emphasizing the need for regular and correct PFME. These midwives need to be regularly updated with new information and encouraged to communicate with one another in the ongoing antenatal and postpartum care of women. Thus, midwives need to be actively involved in educating and demonstrating to pregnant women about SUI during pregnancy and how to perform PFME while encouraging the women to adhere to recommended PFME regimens. The purpose of this chapter is to discuss knowledge about SUI and PFME during pregnancy. This information can be useful for midwives and healthcare professionals when informing and counseling pregnant women in SUI prevention during pregnancy.

In: Midwifery
Editor: Gordon Dennel
ISBN: 978-1-63463-113-6

Chapter 1

TRAINING OF TRADITIONAL MIDWIVES IN ECUADOR AND MEXICO: PROMOTING INCLUSIVENESS OR CULTURAL MARGINALIZATION OF TRADITIONAL MEDICINE?

Maria Costanza Torri
University of New Brunswick, Canada

ABSTRACT

Public health programs in Latin America are encouraging the participation of traditional midwives in trainings programs on birth, delivery practices and risks reduction. Although the existing literature focuses on the health outcomes of training of traditional midwives, there is a paucity of research analyzing the perceptions and the acceptance of such training programs by traditional midwives.

What is the perception of midwives who have been trained vis-à-vis these training programs? Are these training programs an effective way to reduce the marginalization of traditional midwifery and to enhance stronger forms of collaboration between traditional medicinal systems and biomedicine? Or on the contrary are they a way to reinforce the dominance and dependence of traditional midwives towards biomedicine?

This chapter analyzes the way in which training programs in Ecuador and Mexico have transformed the role of traditional midwives and their perceptions of traditional midwifery identity and practices in their process of negotiation between traditional medicine and biomedicine.

Keywords: Ecuador, Mexico, traditional midwives, training programs

INTRODUCTION

The role of traditional midwives varies across cultures and at different times and even today these traditional practitioners attend the majority of deliveries in rural areas in developing countries. According to WHO (2008) each year 45 million births occur at home without skilled health personnel. Skilled attendants assist in more than 99% of births in more developed countries, versus 62% in developing countries.

In many rural and periurban communities, the perinatal care that traditional midwives offer is generally profoundly rooted in the local culture and collectively valuated as the result of hand-on experience. There is little doubt that traditional midwives play an important role when it comes to cultural competence, empathy and psychosocial support at birth with important benefits for the mother and the new-born baby (Cosminsky, 2001).

Since the Alma-Ata conference in 1978, there has been an increase of studies on the characteristics, attitudes and practices of traditional midwifery intended to inform policy action on a possible integration between midwifery and biomedical practices.

The international interest to integrating traditional midwives into national health care systems as a strategy to reduce the high rates of maternal mortality has intensified the pressures of medicalization of midwifery practices in numerous countries in Latin America (Belliard and Ramírez-Johnson, 2005; Cosminsky, 2001). In many countries, such as Mexico and Ecuador, training traditional midwives represents an important strategy to improve maternal and neo-natal outcomes. The goal of traditional midwives' training is to contribute to the decline of maternal mortality and morbidity through better delivery and child care practices by: i) enhancing the skills and knowledge of traditional midwives; ii) increasing the number of births conducted by trained traditional midwives; and iii) improving the relations between biomedical health services and the community through traditional midwives.

But how do the midwives who have been trained perceive these trainings programs? Are these programs able to promote stronger forms of collaboration between traditional midwifery practices and biomedicine? Or quite the contrary, do these training programs reinforce the domination and dependency of traditional midwives towards biomedicine?

By addressing the interaction between the hand-on knowledge of traditional midwives and the biomedical system, this chapter examines biomedical and local beliefs and practices surrounding birth in Mexico and Ecuador, paying particular attention to the issue of training programs of traditional midwives.

Training Programs for Traditional Midwives: Promoting Inclusiveness?

Training programs addressed to traditional midwives are generally designed to teach them about general hygiene and preventive reproductive care, to encourage them to refer pregnant women to the hospital for prenatal examinations, delivery and postpartum follow-up, as well as to teach midwives to identify risk factors during pregnancies (Huber and Sandstrom, 2001; Hurtado and Saenz de Tejada, 2001).

The training programs aiming at strengthening the partnership between traditional midwifery and biomedicine have been criticised (Bailey et al., 2002; Cosminsky, 2001; Goldman and Glei, 2003). The criticisms moved to these programs are that they are unnecessarily complicated and inappropriate for local midwives who are often illiterate. Moreover, the medical staff teaching these training programs does not usually speak indigenous languages. This fact hinders the communication between the stakeholders and makes it difficult for traditional midwives to fully grasp the technical and medical concepts underlying these courses. Besides, these training programs generally use teaching methods that are not culturally inappropriate, encourage the use of procedures often unrealistic in the midwives' settings and discourage traditional practices (e.g., delivery in an upright rather than supine position and traditional massage).

Houston (2000) maintains that the training programs for traditional midwives have most of the time been unable to understand the richness of traditional midwives' knowledge and practices, thus failing to create a respectful and productive working relationship between medical staff and traditional midwives. Traditional practices, such as the use of herbal teas and massage are often condemned while the adoption of biomedical practices is encouraged (Jordan, 1997; Foster et al. 2004). As Hobart (1993) suggests, fundamental to the concept of development is the modernist assumption that it requires the attainment of particular legitimized knowledge, which is progressive and continuous. Attachment to "tradition," to local practices and rituals, is thus constructed as an obstacle to change and as responsible for the continuation of "ignorance" (Hobart 1993).

One can question whether the central focus of these training programs is to undermine traditional midwifery practices and replace them with the biomedical model of health (Feldhusen, 2000, Bailey et al., 2005; Cosminsky, 2001). According to Davis-Floyd (2003: 1916):*'Very seldom do the ''trainers'' enter a community and spend time there learning about indigenous birthways before they try to intervene. Rather, they attempt to educate traditional midwives in biomedical ways of thinking, most especially about conditions of risk that are deemed to necessitate transport'.*

The impact of these trainings on influencing midwifery practices has also been questioned. Although some studies highlight that training has had an impact on traditional knowledge, practices, or referrals (Kumar et al., 2000; Islam and Malik, 2001), others find little or no effect (Smith et al., 2000; Goodburn et al., 2000; Smith et al., 2000).When surveyed on their practices, trained midwives often show almost identical scores to untrained midwives in terms of what medical staff consider "beneficial" and "harmful" practices (Glei and Goldman, 2000; Huber and Sandstrom, 2001).

In order to include traditional midwifery into biomedicine, it is crucial to comprehend the traditional forms of knowledge and practices (Davis-Floyd, 2002; Houston, 2000; Smith et al., 2000). As meanings are profoundly shaped by cultural contexts and individual perceptions, knowledge transfer should consider people's constructions of reality and the meaning they attribute to it (Davis-Floyd, 2002). When this does not happen, knowledge transfer may strengthen hierarchies of knowledge and practices and in some cases promote opposing forms of conflicting knowledge. As reported by critics of expert knowledge transfer (Davis-Floyd, 2003; Penn et al., 1995), knowledge transfer may ignore the fact that social actors, including in this case the traditional midwives, make sense of their world as they interact with others, within a social landscape with multiple realities. Because meanings are embedded in people's visions of reality, which in turn are shaped by cultural contexts, history, religion, and science, knowledge transfer would need to take into account people's meaning and visions of reality. When this is ignored, knowledge transfer may create a situation with a hierarchy of knowledge and practice, but also parallel authoritative or competing knowledge.

Although training in traditional midwifery is now widespread, it is not clear how effective the training programs in enhancing the quality of reproductive care for local women and whether they practically benefit traditional midwives in their practices and how they shape their sense of identity as traditional practitioners.

This study wants to contribute to this research gap by analyzing the ways in which training programs have possibly produced a shift in the perceptions of traditional midwifery identity and in their therapeutic practices in Mexico and Ecuador.

First Case Study: Mexico

In Mexico traditional medical practices such as midwifery, have been often disregarded by the health policy makers till the early 1970s. Till the 70's the main preoccupation was indeed to attain a rapid and pervasive process of 'modernization' of the health care system to be achieved through a form of reliance on biomedicine and modern technology (DeVries et al. 2004, Geurts, 2001, Torres and De Vries, 2009).

In 1972, the Mexican government started the first training programs for traditional midwives (*parteras*) to improve maternal and child care; by 1977, the training included a section on family planning.

In the process of incorporation of midwives by the Mexican government into the institutional health care services, more than 15,000 *parteras* were trained between 1974 and the beginning of the 1980s (Malvarez and Castrillon, 2005). As a result of these changes, it has become both easier and bureaucratically beneficial for *parteras* to attend training classes and receive a license. In fact, only licensed *parteras* can register a newborn, the government requires a licensed midwife's signature and official seal on the birth registration form if the baby is not born at the hospital.

Methodology

The data are based on a fieldwork carried out between February and March 2009 in the state of Tamaulipas, in the town of Tula located in the Tula municipality. Thirty-two in-depth interviews were conducted, seventeen with traditional midwives (*parteras*) and fifteen with pregnant women or with women who already delivered the babies.

Traditional midwives were recruited with the support of health care providers at the local hospital and through local acquaintances. The remaining midwives were recruited through snow-ball sampling. The age of the *parteras* ranged between 48 and 68 years. The traditional midwives varied in terms of schooling: two/thirds of the *parteras* interviewed had between four and five years of schooling and the remaining ones were educated beyond the primary level. The majority of the *parteras* (ten out of seventeen) attended the training courses organized at the hospital on regular basis (ie., every month or every two months).

Semi-structured questions aimed to assess the point of view of the interviewees about the efficacy of biomedical and traditional health practices in midwifery, as well to gain an understanding on the perceptions of midwives on the training programs they attended.

Two group interviews with traditional midwives were also carried out. The twelve traditional midwives who participated in the focus groups were selected from those who participated in the individual interviews, the criteria for the selection being their work experience, number of deliveries and the frequency with which they participated in the governmental training programmes.

Results

Ten of the seventeen *parteras* interviewed had attended training programs recently and all but one of the midwives interviewed had attended a training course at some point in their careers.

More than half of the midwives who have more than 20 years of experience affirmed that they learned their skills and expertise from older midwives. None of them stated that they learned the practice from training programs. This data should be contrasted with the midwives having five or fewer years of experience. Only four midwives included in this category affirmed that they directly learned from other experienced midwives.

The complaints from the *parteras* vis-à-vis training programs focused on the lack of respect for the knowledge and practices of *parteras* and the overarching sentiment of fear and incompetence that many training programs seem to have created among the participants.

In Tula, despite the increasing dominance of the biomedical health care system, older midwives emphasized the importance and the significance of their own knowledge and experience and contextualized the relevance of training programs within their own experiential knowledge and abilities.

Although experienced midwives recognized the value of the training courses, the majority of older midwives affirmed that they already possessed a sufficient understanding of midwifery practice. The new midwives were more influenced by the training programs and the biomedical model served as the template for their own stated practice. Trained and inexperienced midwives reflected the biomedical practices which they learned in training courses in reference with the delivery positions and the reasons for and timing of referrals to the hospital. Interviews with younger midwives (around 40-45 years old) showed how the construction of biomedical training also shaped the value and relevance they attributed to traditional midwifery practices. Young and recently trained midwives constantly attributed their capacity and expertise in midwifery to their participation in training programs and minimized the relevance of the experiential knowledge of older midwives. This attitude is reflected in the statement of a midwife in her early forties who affirmed:

> 'When I started my practice as a midwife I was very preoccupied as I was not sure of myself and I did not know much about this profession. Luckily I attended some training courses organized at the Tula hospital and now I have learnt how to do the work'.

Taking about their experience with biomedical professionals during the training sessions, nine out of seventeen traditional midwives interviewed affirmed that they often felt not at ease in the company of doctors and declared that they felt nervous that the doctors would have undermined their knowledge in front of the patients. This illustrates that the sense of identity of the *parteras* was affected by their interactions with biomedical professionals. While they felt good that they were helping their patients to get quality biomedical care, it resulted in diminished self-esteem because the interactions often made the traditional midwives feel incapable or ashamed.

Second Case Study: Ecuador

The training of traditional midwives and the creation of intercultural, vertical maternity wards were incorporated in the government's strategy.

Considering the experience of San Luis of Otavalo Hospital, the Public Health Ministry of Ecuador is envisaging to implement this practice in other hospitals, nationwide. So far, intercultural maternity centers that incorporate vertical birthing practices have spread from Otavalo to the provinces of Chimborazo, Amazonia and Esmeraldas.

The hospital of San Luis is located in the northern part of the city of Otavalo, in an area of two hectares and was built in 1953. The hospital provides health services of prenatal and postpartum care, delivery care and family planning. The region of Otavalo was described in 2003 as an area in risk of maternal death and neonatal tetanus. In the years between 2001 and 2005, in the region of Otavalo, there were ten cases of maternal death; all deaths happened in the rural area.

The hospital of San Luis began a pilot proposal for the incorporation of the intercultural approach in reproductive health services in April 2008, in order to provide better care for indigenous women who had no access to health care due to cultural barriers. More specifically, the role of midwives within the institutional collaboration with the San Luis hospital consists on the following tasks:

I. Carrying out home visits and counseling on reproductive health during pregnancy for the prompt identification of potential risks during pregnancies,
II. Accompanying the pregnant women to the hospital for checkups during pregnancy,
III. Accompanying pregnant women to the hospital for delivery and helping the medical staff in the delivery process by entering the labor room,
IV. Providing physical support for women in labor with massages,
V. Providing emotional support for women in labor, accompanying and supporting them,
VI. Giving women herbal teas and medicinal plants according to the needs and stages of labor, and in consultation with the professional staff.

Methods

The fieldwork for this study was conducted in Ecuador between May and July of 2011 at San Luis Hospital in the city of Otavalo (Imbabura Province).

Fifty interviews were conducted, ten with traditional midwives (*parteras*) and forty with pregnant women or with women who already delivered the babies. Seven doctors working at the delivery ward at the San Luis hospital of Otavalo as well as eight nurses were interviewed.

Data were collected through semi structured and open-ended interviews, home visits, and observation in homes and in the local hospital of San Luis in Otavalo. The interviewees were selected on the basis of the experience they had developed and the reputation they acquired within the community.

The midwives interviewed had an average age of sixty years (two-thirds of the interviewees), the level of education was generally primary education (half of the interviewees), the other half of them being illiterate.

The interviews, whose duration ranged between 45 minutes to one hour each, consisted of structured and semi-structured components. After previous consent, the interviews have been tape-recorded and subsequently translated in English.

Primary thematic categories were developed and independent coders established reliability in the use of the coding system before all excerpts had been formally analyzed. Data have been summarized thematically and with illustrative quotes to capture the perspectives represented in the interviews.

Results

The majority of the doctors interviewed (i.e., four) declared to be favorable to the presence of *parteras* and affirmed that the *parteras* improved the service offered by the hospital, especially vis-à-vis indigenous communities. Despite this, the majority of the doctors affirmed that the role of *parteras* should have been primarily confined to the psychological realm for the patients the hospital, by playing a role of cultural and linguistic "mediators" with the indigenous patients.

Interviews highlighted how some *parteras*, especially the younger ones, had become interested in learning about allopathic drugs, especially those used to speed up the delivery process, reduce pain during the delivery and the bleeding. The use of these drugs may help midwives appear ''modern'' in a society that looks with approval at signs of modernity among health workers. This aspect is particularly delicate and raises doubts on the possible emergence of risky behaviours, especially if these medications are used without the supervision of a doctor in patients with delicate health conditions (i.e., those suffering from high blood pressure and diabetes).

The interviews with the *parteras* working in the hospital show that there was a process of possible exchange of knowledge between indigenous medicine and biodimecine among midwives and nurses. The *parteras* stated that some nurses were interested in learning the use of native plants and massage and midwives were rather interested in learning more about the use the allopathic medicines. However, when asked the name of the plants used by the *parteras* for reproductive health, only two nurses were able to name some of these plants and their uses. Thus, it seems to be a lack of genuine exchange of knowledge between the medical staff and the *parteras* although the interaction between them seems to have increased their interest in learning more about their mutual practices.

The doctors interviewed affirmed that they learned from the *parteras* how to carry out vertical birth. This practice has been praised by some doctors as being easier for the women and generally allowing a faster delivery of the baby. Other advantages emphasized by the nurses and obstetricians regarding vertical delivery were that the perineal tissues stretched more effectively, often reducing the need for postpartum repairs. This represented a positive aspect of acceptance of traditional knowledge from the biomedical staff at the hospital.

Despite the positive acceptance of this traditional midwifery practice by the biomedical staff at the hospital, a practice such as traditional massage through which the *parteras* were able to redirect the baby in the right position in the mother's womb, thus avoiding a C-section, was generally criticized and defined as dangerous and inappropriate.

This result is consistent with other ethnographic studies of pregnancy and delivery who emphasize the divergence between the biomedical model that dominates the provision of formal health care practices surrounding birth (Bailey et al., 2005; Lorentzen, 2008). This discrepancy is a matter of concern for public health professionals who fear that "traditional culture" may represent an obstacle to health and a potential risk.

CONCLUSION

Public health programs including traditional midwives represent an important initiative to improve reproductive health of local women. Nevertheless, the acceptance of situated forms of knowledge still seems problematic in these programs. Alcoff et al. (1993) use the term “epistemology discrimination” to describe the attitude that produces a form of discrimination between different kinds of knowledge. This produces a lack of recognition between the different types of knowledge, thus preventing an effective exploration and utilisation of the available knowledge.

The case studies analyzed in this chapter indicate that there is a lack of significant exchange and communication between biomedical knowledge and traditional knowledge despite their institutionalized cooperation. The training programs for traditional midwives analyzed in this chapter seem to be limited to transferring the type of knowledge the health system thinks the traditional midwives need to know and not vice versa. This is aggravated by the fact that the biomedical health system has generally a very limited understanding about traditional midwifery or it has decided to overlook it all together.

Despite the fact that training courses for traditional midwives have been promoted in several countries in Latin America, Mexico and Ecuador included, most of these efforts have not attaint the positive expected results. The training programs analyzed in these case studies have not been able to effectively put into value the expertise existing among traditional midwives. When traditional midwives attend training programmes they are supposed to incorporate in their knowledge what "modern" health practitioners are supposed to do and say. This biomedical knowledge is perceived as "authoritative" by the traditional midwives not because it is presented as such by the medical staff but because training comes out of institutions, such as hospitals, that are authoritatively representing the "developed" world overall. Training programmes thus can amplify the sense of disparity among traditional midwives between "modern" practices and their devalued and "outdated" local realities.

The training programs for traditional midwives deliver a biomedical ideology not just through their specific technical content but also through the insistence in their format that the physiological aspects should be clearly separated from social and religious concerns. Thus, the biomedical ideology, implicitly passed through training, requires trainees themselves to fragment their practices, to distinguish between the "medical" and the "social" aspects of what they do.

The complex relationship between discourse and power is a dominant aspect in all of this because any exercise of power by human beings is influenced by the discursive nature of power itself (Foucault (1980). Corson (2000) maintained that the conflict that takes place around discourse can be biased if the balance of power constantly favours some group while discriminating others. This can be seen in the obstetric versus midwifery discourse presented in the choices and procedures in the training programs which ensure the ideological dominance of biomedicine and which serve to silence midwives (McCall, 1996; Farrell, 1997)

Although this chapter analyzed some of the challenges of integrating traditional midwifery practices with biomedicine, the positive outcomes of the collaboration between midwives and biomedical practitioners cannot be underestimated. Professionalizing midwifery and complementing it with medical approaches could allow reduce the risks of childbirth and improve the health outcomes of mothers and their newborn babies, especially in rural areas.

The existing training programs promoting the integration of traditional midwives with the biomedical health system provide a space to explore two knowledge systems put together for a common cause. i.e., improve the quality of health services. Training programs for traditional midwives have a potential to improve the quality of reproductive health, this important goal should be accomplished while fully respecting the local cultural values. Indeed, it is vital to promote training programs that challenge the existing model and that are capable of producing more than just formal changes in the future collaboration between traditional medicine and biomedicine. Training programmes should critically examine the basis upon which they are developed and begin to move from a hierarchical model to one that is more egalitarian. Programs should acknowledge the potential of midwives to engage in social action and social change and recognize the fact that midwifery is more than just transmitting anatomy and physiology or helping to give birth.

In conclusion, it is critical to set up training programs as well as strategies for promoting healthy relationships between traditional midwives and the biomedical health care system, as well as to provide traditional midwives with continuous support and respect. In order to comprehend someone's perspective on health and therapeutic practices, it is important to understand their background and experience. Overlooking midwives' voice and denying their experience can undermine the richness of the midwife's knowledge and the understanding of her expertise in reproductive health.

Unless the transfer of knowledge through training is based on the understanding and recognition of the contexts and realities of the people concerned, it is hard to envisage any success. The case studies analyzed show the importance of promoting an approach that integrates traditional knowledge and recognises multiple realities, with a view of giving voice to stakeholders of different perspectives, including those who are normally ignored or left out.

REFERENCES

Alcoff, L. (1993). Feminist Epistemologies. London, Routledge.

Bailey, P., E. de Bocaletti, G. Barrios, and Y. de Cross, (2002). Monitoring Utilization and Need for Obstetric Care in the Highlands of Guatemala. International Journal of Gynecology and Obstetrics, 8(9):209-217.

Belliard, J., Ramírez-Johnson, J., (2005). Medical Pluralism in the Life of a Mexican Migrant Woman. Hispanic Journal of Behavioral Sciences, 2(7): 267-285.

Cosminsky, S. (2001). Maya Midwives of Southern Mexico and Guatemala. In Mesoamerican Healers. Brad R. Huber and Alan R. Sandstrom, eds. Pp. 179-210 Austin, TX: University of Texas Press.

Davis-Floyd, R. (2003).Home-birth emergencies in the US and Mexico: the trouble with transport, Social Science & Medicine, 5(6):1911-1931.

Davis-Floyd, R. (2002). Anthropological perspectives on global issues in midwifery, Midwifery Today, 2002, 1–12.

DeVries, R. (2004). A Pleasing Birth: Midwives and Maternity Care in the Netherlands. Philadelphia: Temple University Press.

Farrell, A. (1997). Aggression in clinical settings: nurses' view. Journal of Advanced Nursing 25: 50 1-508.

Foster, J., Anderson, A., Houston, J. Doe-Simkins, M. (2004). A Midwifery Model for Training Traditional Midwives in Guatemala: A Report from the Field. Midwifery, 20(3), 217-225.

Foucault, M. (1980). Truth and Power. In Power/Knowledges: Selected Interviews and Other Writings 1972-77, edited by C. Gordon, 109-133. New York: Pantheon.

Geurts, K. (2001). Childbirth and Pragmatic Midwifery in Rural Ghana. Medical Anthropology, 20(2-3):45-52.

Glei, D. A., Goldman, N. (2000). Understanding Ethnic Variation in Pregnancy-Related Health Care in Rural Guatemala. Ethnicity and Health, 5(1), 5-22.

Goldman, N., Glei, D. A. (2003). Evaluation of midwifery care: Results from a survey in rural Guatemala. Social Science & Medicine, 5(6), 685-700.

Goodburn, E. A., Chowdhury, M., Gazi, R., Marshall, T., Graham, W. (2000). Training traditional birth attendants in clean delivery doesnot prevent postpartum infection. Health Policy and Planning, 15(4), 394-399.

Hobart, M. (1993). Introduction: the Growth of Ignorance? In An Anthropological Critique of Development: The Growth of Ignorance. M. Hobart, ed. Pp. 1-30. London: Routledge.

Huber, B. R., Sandstrom, A. R. (2001). Recruitment, training, and practice of indigenous midwives: From the Mexico–United States border to the Isthmus of Tehuantepec. In B. R. Huber, & A. R. Sandstrom (Eds.), Mesoamerican healers (pp. 139–178). Austin: University of Texas Press.

Hurtado, E., Saenz de Tejada, E. (2001). Relations between government health workers and traditional midwives in Guatemala. In B. R. Huber, & A. R. Sandstrom (Eds.), Mesoamerican healers (pp. 211–242). Austin: University of Texas Press.

Houston, J. (2000). Weaving a Cultural Exchange: Midwives Working Together. Midwifery Today, 5(3), 34-35.

Islam, A., Malik, F. A. (2001). Role of traditional birth attendants in improving reproductive health: Lessons from the family health project, Sindh. *Journal of the Pakistan Medical Association*, 51(6), 218-222.

Jordan, B. (1997). Authoritative knowledge and its construction. In R. E. Davis-Floyd, & C. F. Sargent (Eds.). Childbirth and authoritative knowledge (pp. 55–79). Berkeley, Los Angeles, London: University of California Press.

Kumar, R., Thakur, J. S., Aggarwal, A. K. (2000). Effect of continuing training on knowledge and practices of traditional birth attendants about maternal and newborn care. *Indian Journal of Public Health*, 44(4), 118-123.

Lorentzen, J. M. (2008). I Know My Own Body': Power and Resistance in Women's Experiences of Medical Interactions. Body and Society, 14(49):49-79.

Malvarez S., Castrillon, C. (2005). Overview of the nursing workforce in Latin America. Human Resources Development Series No.39. Washington DC7 PAHO.

McCall, E. (1996). Horizontal Violence in Nursing: The Continuing Silence. The Lamp, April: 28-30.

Penn, N. Kar, J., Skimmer, J. Zambrana, R. (1995). *Ethnic minorities, health care system and behaviour, Health Psychology,* 1(4): 641-656.

Smith, J. B., Coleman, N. A., Fortney, J. A., Johnson, J. D., Blumhagen, D. W., Grey, T. W. (2000). The impact of traditional birth attendant training on delivery complications in Ghana. *Health Policy and Planning*, 15(3), 326-331.

Torres, J. M., De Vries, R. (2009). Birthing Ethics: What Mothers, Families, Childbirth Educators, Nurses, and Physicians Should Know About the Ethics of Childbirth. *Journal of Perinatal Education,* 18(1), 2-24.

In: Midwifery
Editor: Gordon Dennel

ISBN: 978-1-63463-113-6

Chapter 2

How Can We Teach Midwifery Students to Become Caring Midwives?

Sigfridur Inga Karlsdottir* and Sigridur Halldorsdottir
School of Health Sciences, University of Akureyri, Akureyri, Iceland

Abstract

Midwives are a key profession in the care of women during the childbearing process, and research results indicate that they can have a major effect upon their wellbeing and health as well as upon their attitude to future births and to their new born child. Women's need for *caring* in the childbearing process and the great importance of the *caring midwife* has been established by listening, through research, to women who have given birth. The detrimental effects of uncaring has also been demonstrated in the same way. What is caring then? What is uncaring? How can we recognize and avoid uncaring? More importantly, how can we teach caring and how can we help midwifery students to avoid being perceived as uncaring? Finally, how should midwifery education be organized in order to educate caring midwives? These are the basic questions we will try to answer in this discussion paper. We conclude that during revision of midwifery education programmes the focus should always be on how all the different aspects of the complicated project of educating a "good midwife" be included in the curriculum and that the importance of caring will not be left out.

* Corresponding author: School of Health Sciences, University of Akureyri, Solborg, P.O. Box, 224, 602 Akureyri, Iceland, E-mail: inga@unak.is.

The Great Importance of the Caring Midwife

Caring midwives and how important they are in women's birth experiences has been clear to us ever since our first studies in 1996. The women in our studies have seen their *birth experience as a journey* (Halldorsdottir & Karlsdottir, 1996a) and have described the caring midwives as *indispensable companions* on the journey through labor and delivery (Halldorsdottir & Karlsdottir, 1996b).

What then is *caring in midwifery*? The women in our research have described the caring midwives as able to give of themselves, able to show solidarity and share the birth experience with the woman, encouraging and supportive, respectful and benevolent, cheerful and positive, reliable and trustworthy, considerate and understanding. They also saw the midwives' *professional competence* as a part of *professional caring* because the midwives perceived as truly caring were also described as competent; having the necessary knowledge and skills needed to coach a woman through the journey of labor and delivery; responsible, attentive, deliberate and able to communicate effectively. Such a caring midwife, they felt, was committed in safeguarding their personal integrity and dignity. The women felt that this caring midwife made them feel connected, safe and at ease, as well as being able to be herself on her journey through labor and delivery.

Unfortunately, our study and that of others (Eliasson, Kainz, & von Post, 2008; Halldorsdottir & Karlsdottir, 1996a) indicate that women do not always experience midwives as caring and can even find some of them discouraging and uncaring. They described the midwife perceived as uncaring as thoughtless, strict on routine and rules, not taking notice of the woman and the women described lack of co-operation and a sense of togetherness. They also described the midwives perceived as uncaring as indifferent and untouched by the event as such, lacking in interest and understanding in general, non-supportive and insensitive, as well as a tendency to be hurried and in a rush. They also described the midwives perceived as uncaring as gloomy and brusque, cold, unkind and harsh. The women also described the midwives perceived as uncaring as lacking in competence; rough when giving care to the woman, ineffective in communication, not taking initiative when needed and lacking in understanding as well as lacking flexibility. In our research the women have related that uncaring in their sensitive situation had negative effects on them. Their first reaction seemed to be one of puzzlement and disbelief and an effort in trying to make sense of the uncaring. Experiencing an encounter with a midwife perceived as uncaring left the women feeling unconnected and alone as well as feeling abandoned in a vulnerable situation. The uncaring midwife was perceived as *an unfortunate hindrance to a successful birth experience* (Halldorsdottir & Karlsdottir, 1996a) and in many cases the bitter experience had negative long-term consequences, as this account shows:

> "I felt very insecure throughout this whole period and I felt that I.. and I didn´t feel in good hands. I felt that I .. I somehow felt that I was stuck with all the responsibility. That was not a comfortable feeling. I promised myself after this that I would not go through more births and I have kept that promise. Never in my whole life would I go through a birth again! (p. 374).

This has been confirmed in a later study that a negative birth experience can influence women's decisions about subsequent childbearing (Gottwall & Waldenström, 2002). We can therefore see that the midwife can have tremendous effects on the woman on her journey through labor and delivery.

We have continued to listen to women about their birth experiences because we see *the perspective of childbearing women* as representing an important '*third paradigm in midwifery care*' (Karlsdottir, Halldorsdottir, & Lundgren, 2013); the first and second being the midwifery and the medical paradigm, respectively. We have developed our ideas through listening to more childbearing women and we have proposed that professionalism in midwifery is constructed from five main aspects: professional competence, professional wisdom, the midwife's own self-development, interpersonal competence and last but not least the midwife's professional caring (Halldorsdottir & Karlsdottir, 2011). These aspects are all interrelated and are demonstrated in *figure 1.*

The term 'competence' is often used as an umbrella concept covering knowledge, skill, attitudes and the experience required to fulfil a certain role. Certain factors are often cited as requirements for a specified field of work. In an evolving theory of professionalism in midwifery (Halldorsdottir & Karlsdottir, 2011) the five above-mentioned aspects are seen as the basis of professionalism in midwifery: Professional caring, professional competence, professional wisdom, interpersonal competence and the midwife's self-development (see *table 2*).

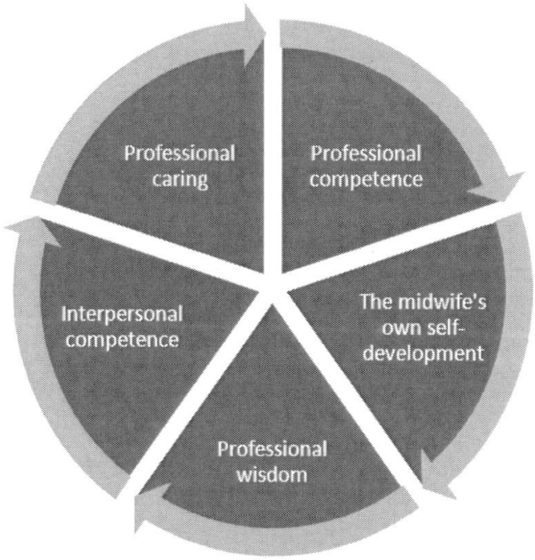

Figure 1. An overview of the main aspects of professionalism in midwifery (Based on Halldorsdottir & Karlsdottir, 2011).

If any of these important factors is lacking, the service is incomplete in some way and can have a *discouraging effects* on the woman journeying through labor and delivery. We assert that a professional midwife who is caring and professionally competent and who has interpersonal skills and professional wisdom is a *good midwife*. A good midwife is in many ways like a personal guide, who leads the woman and her family through the journey of the childbearing process and whose guidance is adapted to the needs of each woman and her family. We maintain that a caring midwife utilizes all communications to strengthen the woman, for instance by providing information and the appropriate knowledge. The influence of the encounter with a good midwife is best described as *empowerment*. We are aware that empowerment is a term that has been open to critique. Our understanding of empowerment is that the midwife "strengthens a woman's confidence facilitating recognition of her own strengths and capacities." (Halldorsdottir & Karlsdottir, 2011, p. 811).

In our view, midwifery service based on *the childbearing women's perspective* is always based on professional caring and the wish to increase the health and well-being of childbearing women where each woman is seen as a unique individual with the right to maintain dignity and to use her own resources to manage through the childbearing process. How then can we educate midwifery students to be caring midwives?

Table 1. An overview of the good midwife's professionalism (Halldorsdottir & Karlsdottir, 2011)

THE MIDWIFE'S PROFESSIONALISM encompasses five main aspects:	DESCRIPTION OF THE ESSENTIAL ASPECT
1. Professional caring	The midwife cares for the woman and her family. This *individualized caring* is the *heart of midwifery* from the childbearing women's perspective.
2. Professional wisdom	The midwife has *wisdom* and knows how to apply it within midwifery. Such wisdom develops through *the interplay of knowledge and experience*.
3. Professional competence	The midwife is competent and this *competence has primacy in midwifery to ensure the safety of mother and child*.
4. Interpersonal competence	The midwife is capable of *empowering communication* and *partnership* with the woman and her family. For many women, *this partnership is the difference between perceived caring and uncaring*.
5. The midwife's personal and professional development	The midwife knows and nurtures herself, both personally and professionally which prevents her burnout.

THE PERSPECTIVE OF MIDWIFERY STUDENTS

Studies have been conducted to explore midwifery students' view on midwifery education and according to results of a study conducted among final year midwifery students in Australia the *passion for midwifery* and *continuing determination* were seen as important parts of personal traits during midwifery education (Carolan-Olah, Kruger, Walter, & Mazzarino, 2013). Result from another study performed in the Netherlands indicates that midwifery students identify two types of care, named '*factory-style care*' and '*tailored care*'. Participants in that study linked 'style of care' more to a person than to a profession and according to the results it is different what ideology people adhere to and what attitude they have towards to childbearing women (Van kelst, Spitz, Sermeus, & Thomson, 2013). Thus, they state that although 'women-centered ideology' during their education is adhered to during midwifery education that is not always the reality and that students should learn about differences in styles of care and how to deal with them.

In a study by Schytt and Waldenström (2013) several items are measured to identify midwifery student's view on how well they are prepared for clinical practice. The results show that most of the students were satisfied with how the education prepared them for clinical practice. The authors emphasize that midwives today need to be more clinically competent than before, because of medical technologies that have become a part of clinical work in midwifery in the last decades.

Furthermore, technology has made it possible to detect and act on signs of complications that were not possible before. We agree that technology is important for example to maximize the likelihood of safe childbirth but on the other hand professions like midwives must remember that there are also other competencies that are important if we want to provide professional care during childbirth care in the manner that the childbearing woman feels cared for.

Study conducted in Australia among midwifery students researching their view regarding the role of midwives indicates that they experience the job as 'complicated' where they had to combine being *a skilled practitioner*, *a caring and compassionate individual* and frequently go *beyond the call of duty* (Carolan, 2011). Those themes indicate that midwifery students experience midwifery as a profession where different skills are needed to become a good midwife. But how can we teach midwifery student to become a "good midwives".

Educating Midwifery Students to be Caring Midwives

If we want to provide good midwifery education we have to be able to address difficult topics such as when women journeying through labor and delivery do not experience midwives as caring. In our study, an uncaring midwife was seen by the women as someone who lacks, for example, respect for women and is rough when giving care to women or lacks genuine concern for the woman as a person. The effects of encounters with a midwife perceived as uncaring seem to be a sense of *being discouraged* and *feeling abandoned* and *frustrated*.

Women have also indicated that those effects can be long lasting and bitter experiences in their lives as mothers and persons in their coming future. On the other hand, the experience of a caring encounter with a midwife gives the woman a sense of being empowered by their midwife and the feeling of trust, safety and a feeling of a successful birth even though it is a long and difficult one (Halldorsdottir & Karlsdottir, 1996a). Women's descriptions of caring and uncaring are therefore very important in midwifery education. The key differences are portrayed in *table 2* and can be used as guiding lights in the teaching about caring and how to avoid being perceived as uncaring.

We have not come across a study on caring and uncaring encounters with teachers from the perspective of midwifery students but in such a study from nursing students' perspective they explicitly emphasized that *caring* was one of the most important aspects of a good professional teacher in their experience. From their perspective they saw caring as genuine concern for students, being attentive to the individual student and being interested in the student's future, having respect for students and being concerned that they really learn, as well as having faith in students as studying persons. The former students also emphasized the teacher's professional competence, positive personality and professional commitment as well as being able to connect with students. Because of the positive teacher-student connection the former students experienced a *positive working relationship* with the teachers perceived as professional and caring. The former students described how much they appreciated the caring teachers and described their desire to model themselves after them.

The former students seemed to internalize the teacher's values and outlook in a considerable way which often resulted in *a positive image of their profession and themselves as professionals* (Halldorsdottir, 1990).

In the same study the students described encounters with teachers perceived to be uncaring and they were perceived to be lacking in professional caring; lacking in professional competence, lacking in concern for the students; demanding control and power and demonstrating destructive behavior. The former students experienced lack of trust in the teachers, perceived as uncaring, as well as a teacher-student detachment with total distance between teacher and student. They found the teachers perceived as uncaring as *demoralizing*.

Table 2. The essential structure of caring and uncaring in midwifery (Based on Halldorsdottir & Karlsdottir, 1996a)

THE ESSENTIAL STRUCTURE OF CARING IN MIDWIFERY: The childbearing woman's perspective	**THE ESSENTIAL STRUCTURE OF UNCARING IN MIDWIFERY: The childbearing woman's perspective**
DESCRIPTION OF CARING: The caring midwives are described as able to give of themselves, able to show solidarity and share the birth experience with the woman, able to be encouraging and supportive, respectful and benevolent, cheerful and positive, reliable and trustworthy, considerate and understanding. Such a caring midwife, they felt, was committed to safeguarding their personal integrity and dignity as women journeying through labor and delivery.	DESCRIPTION OF UNCARING: The uncaring midwives are described as thoughtless, strict on routine and rules, not taking notice of the woman and the women described their lack of co-operation with the woman. They also described the midwives perceived as uncaring as indifferent and untouched by the event as such, lacking in interest and understanding in general, non-supportive and insensitive, as well as being hurried and in a rush. They also described the midwives perceived as uncaring as gloomy and brusque, cold, unkind and harsh.
THE CONNECTION BETWEEN CARING AND COMPETENCE: The women saw the midwives' *professional competence* as a part of *professional caring* because the midwives perceived as truly caring were also described as very competent; having the necessary knowledge and skills needed to coach a woman through the journey of labor and delivery; responsible, attentive, deliberate and able to communicate effectively.	THE CONNECTION BETWEEN UNCARING AND LACK OF COMPETENCE: The women described the midwives perceived as uncaring as also lacking in competence; rough when giving care to the woman, ineffective in communication, not taking initiative when needed and lacking in understanding as well as lacking flexibility.
HOW CARING MADE THE WOMEN FEEL: The women felt that the caring midwives made them feel connected, safe and at ease, as well as being able to be themselves on their journey through labor and delivery. The caring midwives are perceived as *indispensable companions on the journey through labor and delivery.*	HOW UNCARING MADE THE WOMEN FEEL: In our research the women have related that uncaring in their sensitive situation, as women giving birth, had negative effect on them. Experiencing an uncaring encounter with a midwife perceived as uncaring left the women feeling unconnected and alone as well as feeling abandoned in a vulnerable situation. The uncaring midwives were perceived as *an unfortunate hindrance to a successful birth experience.*

We conclude from this study and from others that came after that study that the best way to educate caring midwives is to have *caring midwifery teachers*; teachers who model caring and genuine concern for people, students as well as clients; teachers who are professional, are genuinely concerned for midwifery students, have a positive personality and are professionally committed to midwifery. We are not alone in the conclusion that *a quality teacher is a caring teacher.* On the website of the National Education Association is it written: "showing students you care about them helps create a positive, supportive relationship and helps build an environment where learning can flourish. And you're modeling behavior that you want students to learn and emulate." What does all this mean for midwifery education?

What Does This Mean for Midwifery Education?

Looking at midwifery education worldwide it is important to look at standards for the education. Midwifery education is ultimately important for women's health globally and, therefore, it must be carefully decided upon what should be a part of midwifery education and what not. Professions base their education upon specific objectives of the discipline. Midwifery is such a profession. The objective is to prepare prospective midwives for work in a modern society, within a scholarly discipline, which is also a practice discipline in constant evolution. In our view, curriculum frameworks, theories and models regarding professionalism in midwifery should always include emphasis on *professional caring* and *interpersonal competence* and *the midwife's self-development*, in addition to the *professional competence* required in order to provide a safe service (Halldorsdottir & Karlsdottir, 2011). Hence special attention should be paid to these factors in curriculum planning. Emphasis should be placed upon evaluating the attitudes, interpersonal competence and self-care of student midwives, and not only their cognitive and practical competencies.

The International Confederation of Midwives will celebrate their 100 years anniversary in 2019. The first meeting being recorded in Belgium shortly after the First World War ended. Ever since then midwives have had a formal global cooperation deciding together what midwifery is and what a good midwife stands for. Today midwives from 108 countries participate in the confederation. Every three years the confederation holds a conference and meetings are held where the Confederation Council discusses policy and updates core documents such as guidelines and midwifery standards

(International Confederation of Midwives, 2014). Protocols have been published for what a midwife should be doing and what qualifications are needed as an entry to practice. Such standards also include shared values on which the members of the profession agree. When professional standards are formulated for a profession, these are often minimum standards. Protocols for maternity care have in recent years become more common, and this is to be welcomed, since such guidelines increase evidence based practice.

According to the International Confederation of Midwives, a midwife is a person: who has successfully completed a midwifery education programme that is duly recognized in the country where it is located and that is based on the ICM Essential Competencies for Basic Midwifery Practice and the framework of the ICM Global Standards for Midwifery Education; who has acquired the requisite qualifications to be registered and/or legally licensed to practice midwifery and use the title midwife and who demonstrates competency in the practice of midwifery (International Confederation of Midwives, 2014). Furthermore, the International Confederation of Midwives has developed standards for the scope of practice where working *with women in partnership* is stressed and that a midwife should be a responsible and an accountable professional who gives necessary support, care and advice during pregnancy, labour and the postpartum period (International Confederation of Midwives, 2014).

Within the midwifery society the *partnership with the woman* is highly valued. For example the American College of Nurse-Midwives has the slogan, *with women, for a lifetime* (American College of Nurse-Midwives, 2014). On their webpage the philosophy of care is presented and demonstrated that the power and strength of women are highly valued for the benefit of health and well-being of families, communities and nations. Thus it is acknowledged that every woman has the right to have individual care where her personal strength and her wishes are valued and where her human rights, her right to active participation and her right to maintain own human dignity is appraised. It is also noted that the best models of care are those that promote *a continuous and compassionate partnership*, *acknowledge a person's life experiences* and *involve therapeutic use of a human presence* and *skilful communication* (American College of Nurse-Midwives, 2014).

We should ask ourselves what kind of midwifery education is needed to extend professionalism in the above-mentioned five main aspects of professional midwifery: professional caring, professional competence, professional wisdom, the midwife's own self-development and interpersonal competence (Halldorsdottir & Karlsdottir, 2011). How should a curriculum for midwifery education look like so that midwifery students could at the time they graduate offer such care for women and their families that they are perceived as caring? What kind of knowledge is needed to be a caring and competent midwife that can provide such "optimal health care" for ever women and her family?

Midwives are a key profession in the care of women during the childbearing process, and research results indicate that they can have a major effect upon their wellbeing and their attitude to their new born child (Halldorsdottir & Karlsdottir, 1996a). It is therefore important that during revision of midwifery education programme the focus is always on how the curriculum threads can encompass all the different aspects of the complicated project of educating a 'good midwife'.

Authors have pointed out that medical technology has become a bigger part of clinical work in midwifery in the last decades (Schytt & Waldenström, 2013). It is obvious that more and more time in midwifery education is spent on teaching skills that can be linked to technology and less time to teach other things that are also important. All midwives and midwifery students have to be aware of that danger because at the same time as midwifery students become more and more technically competent less effort may be spent on preparing them in other aspects regarding the profession such as regarding caring.

When planning midwifery education "the theory of the good midwife" can be used to plan what competencies should be taught. How protocols and standards according to the International Confederation of Midwives are met, how much time is spent on each aspect and what kind of skills is taught during the education can be decided upon within that framework. Midwifery teachers can also use the theory as a framework for evaluating competence. Student midwives can use the theory in order to gain a better understanding of what is required of a professional midwife, and the personal qualities they need to nurture in order to become midwives perceived as caring. The theory could also be used to design evaluation forms for assessing student midwives from year to year, and on graduation.

Professional standards in midwifery must be constantly reviewed, and must be in accordance with the latest available knowledge within the profession, and especially studies on women's good and bad experiences of midwifery service. It makes sense to conclude that this is the best way to ensure that midwifery service is in accordance with the wishes and needs of women in the childbearing process. Overemphasis on the importance of science and technology must not hamper midwives expressions of caring.

Midwives and midwifery students must remember at all times what they stand for.

CONCLUSION

Childbearing women's perspective on caring and uncaring encounters with midwives should be part of midwifery education. Teaching midwifery students how all aspects of professional midwifery are linked together and the importance of providing quality care for women and their families is a challenge for all who teach midwifery students how to become caring midwives. We conclude that it is very important to address caring in midwifery education. Midwifery students learn much about antenatal, intra-partum and postnatal care and sometimes it can be complicated to link together knowledge, values and psychomotor skills and provide services based on professional caring. It is, therefore, important to address different aspects of professional caring when teaching midwifery students. Although our modern technological world appears to confront us with an unavoidable trade-off between competence and caring, a progressive view of professional midwifery is that *both competence and caring is required to guide midwifery's art and science*.

REFERENCES

American College of Nurse-Midwives. (2014). Our philosophy of care. Retrieved 19/05/2014 from www.midwife.org/Our-Philosophy-of-Care

Carolan, M. (2011). The good midwife: Commencing students' views. *Midwifery*, *27*(4), 503-508.

Carolan-Olah, M., Kruger, G., Walter, R. & Mazzarino, M. (2013). Final year students' experiences of the bachelor of midwifery course. *Midwifery*.

Eliasson, M., Kainz, G. & von Post, I. (2008). Uncaring midwives. *Nursing Ethics*, *15*(4), 500-511. doi:10.1177/0969733008090521

Gottwall, K. & Waldenström, U. (2002). Does a traumatic birth experience have an impact on future reproduction? *BJOG: International Journal of Obstetrics and Gynaecology*, *109*, 254-260.

Halldorsdottir, S. (1991). Five basic modes of being with another. In D.A. Gaut & M. M. Leininger (Eds.), *Caring: The compassionate healer*. New York: NLN.

Halldorsdottir, S. (1990). The essential structure of a caring and an uncaring encounter with a teacher: The perspective of the nursing student. In M. Leininger & J. Watson (Eds.), *The caring imperative in education*. New York, NY: National League for Nursing.

Halldorsdottir, S. (1997). Implications of the caring/competence dichotomy. In S.E. Thorne & W. E. Hayes (Eds.), *Nursing praxis: Knowledge and action* (pp. 105-124). Thousand Oaks: SAGE.

Halldorsdottir S. & Karlsdottir, S.I. (1996a). Empowerment or discouragement: Women's experience of caring and uncaring encounters during childbirth. *Health Care for Women International*, *17*, 361-377.

Halldorsdottir S. & Karlsdottir, S.I. (1996b). Journeying through labour and delivery: Perceptions of women who have given birth. *Midwifery*, *12*, 48-61.

Halldorsdottir, S. & Karlsdottir, S. I. (2011). The primacy of the good midwife in midwifery services: An evolving theory of professionalism in midwifery. *Scandinavian Journal of Caring Sciences*, *25*, 806-817. Doi:10.1111/j.1471-6712.2011.00886.x

International confederation of midwives. (2014). Retrieved 19/05/14, 2014, Retrieved from www.internationalmidwives.org

Karlsdottir, S. I., Halldorsdottir, S. & Lundgren, I. (2013). The third paradigm in labour pain preparation and management: The childbearing woman's paradigm. *Scandinavian Journal of Caring Sciences*, *28*(2), 315-327. doi:10.1111/scs.12061

National Education Association (NEA) (n.d.). A quality teacher is a caring teacher. The official webpage of NEA. Retrieved from http://www.nea.org/ tools/15751.htm.

Schytt, E. & Waldenström, U. (2013). How well does midwifery education prepare for clinical practice? exploring the views of swedish students, midwives and obstetricians. *Midwifery*, *29*(2), 102-109.

Van kelst, L., Spitz, B., Sermeus, W. & Thomson, A. M. (2013). Student midwives' views on maternity care just before their graduation. *Journal of Advanced Nursing*, *69*(3), 600-609.

In: Midwifery
Editor: Gordon Dennel
ISBN: 978-1-63463-113-6

Chapter 3

PREVENTION AND TREATMENT OF STRESS URINARY INCONTINENCE DURING PREGNANCY: GLOBAL PERSPECTIVE, RESEARCH TO PRACTICE

Bussara Sangsawang, RN, MNS
and Nucharee Sangsawang, RN, MNS
Department of Obstetrics and Gynecological Nursing, Faculty of Nursing, Srinakharinwirot University, Bangkok, Thailand

ABSTRACT

Stress urinary incontinence (SUI), the complaint of involuntary loss of urine on effort, physical exertion, sneezing or coughing, is the most common type of urinary incontinence (UI) in pregnant women. The prevalence of SUI during pregnancy is reported by approximately 18.6% to 75% of all pregnant women.

It is well known that SUI is related to reduced muscle strength, as well as the supportive and sphincteric function of the pelvic floor such as the pelvic floor muscles (PFM), connective tissue and fascia. Pregnancy is one of the main risk factors for the development of SUI. The physiological changes during pregnancy may lead to reduced strength of supportive and sphincteric function of the PFM.

SUI in pregnant women can be prevented and improved by intensive pelvic floor muscle exercise (PFME).

Pregnant women who regularly and correctly perform PFME will have hypertrophy of muscle fibers with strengthening of the PFM and periurethral muscles leading to improvement of the sphincteric function efficiency and decreased urine leakage.

However, some physicians suggest that intensive exercise by a therapist cannot be implemented into clinical practice. It is likely that the success of randomized controlled trials reported in the many research cannot be repeated in a `real clinical situation'.

Most pregnant women tend to consider SUI a common discomfort of pregnancy. Although they are often inconvenienced and troubled by SUI symptoms, they are reluctant to seek help from health professionals. The majority of pregnant women are not provided with information on SUI. During pregnancy, 55% percent of women receive some form of instruction in PFME. This means that not all pregnant women receive instruction about SUI and PFME during pregnancy.

Moreover, the information is provided by a variety of health professionals and no single profession appears to undertake the responsibility of providing this service. Thus, it is suggested that midwives may not have a direct responsibility to provide this knowledge to pregnant women despite the fact that nurses or midwives are health professionals most closely involved with most pregnant women.

Thus, to be effective in the prevention and treatment SUI during pregnancy by PFME, there is a need for the service to be reorganized to ensure that all pregnant women receive high-quality instruction during pregnancy. Midwives should assess the SUI symptoms in pregnant women and provide instruction about SUI and PFME during pregnancy in addition to emphasizing the need for regular and correct PFME.

These midwives need to be regularly updated with new information and encouraged to communicate with one another in the ongoing antenatal and postpartum care of women. Thus, midwives need to be actively involved in educating and demonstrating to pregnant women about SUI during pregnancy and how to perform PFME while encouraging the women to adhere to recommended PFME regimens.

The purpose of this chapter is to discuss knowledge about SUI and PFME during pregnancy. This information can be useful for midwives and healthcare professionals when informing and counseling pregnant women in SUI prevention during pregnancy.

INTRODUCTION

This chapter is aimed at discussing knowledge about stress urinary incontinence and pelvic floor muscle exercise during pregnancy.

Related literature and research papers are explained as presented in the following four parts:

I Stress urinary incontinence during pregnancy.
II Pelvic floor muscle exercise to prevent and treat stress urinary incontinence during pregnancy.
III Factors related to increased compliance with performance of pelvic floor muscle exercise during pregnancy.
IV Role of midwives in promoting pregnant women in the prevention and treatment of stress urinary incontinence during pregnancy.

Part I: Stress Urinary Incontinence during Pregnancy

Urinary incontinence (UI) is defined by the International Continence Society [ICS] as "the complaint of involuntary loss of urine" [1].

Stress urinary incontinence (SUI) is also defined by the ICS as "the complaint of involuntary loss of urine on effort or physical exertion or sneezing or coughing" [1]. Stress urinary incontinence is the most common type of urinary incontinence in women during pregnancy.

Normal Structure and Function of the Lower Urinary Tract

This chapter describes the normal structure and function of the lower urinary tract before describing the pathophysiological mechanisms of SUI. Any understanding of stress incontinence must begin with an accurate appreciation of the detailed anatomy of the continence mechanism and the pelvic floor [2].

The stress continence system includes not only the pelvic floor muscle, but also the sphincteric closure mechanism consisting of urethral striated muscle, urethral smooth muscle and vascular elements with the remainder of the bladder support system consisting of the anterior vagina, endopelvic fascia and bony pelvis [3].

In females, the structure of the lower urinary tract includes the bladder and the female urethra.

Urinary Bladder

Normal continence in women is a complex coordination between the bladder, urethra, pelvic floor muscle and surrounding connective tissue.

Storage of urine is under voluntary control and modulated by the pontine micturition center [4].

The urinary bladder is a hollow muscular organ located in front of the vagina which has two principal functions, namely, to act as a low-pressure reservoir for the storage of urine, and to generate sufficiently high pressure for the expulsion of urine.

The bladder is a highly distensible organ. The lowest part of the bladder is the trigone, which is histologically and embryologically different from the rest to the bladder and contains a rich plexus of neuronal tissue.

The remainder of the bladder is composed of three distinct layers: the serosa which forms the outer adventitial connective tissue layer; detrusor muscle consisting of a smooth muscle layer comprising a randomly arranged syncytium of interlacing muscle bundles; and the urothelium which is an impervious inner layer lined by the transitional cell epithelium [5].

Normal bladder capacity averages 500-600 ml. The urinary bladder must function as a low pressure expandable reservoir to maintain continence, i.e. the pressure within the bladder must remain lower than the urethral pressure [5, 6].

Urethra

The female urethra is the lower continuation of the bladder located behind the symphysis pubis and in front of the vagina. The female urethra has two functions: to provide an effective continence mechanism during urine storage and to facilitate emptying from the bladder with minimum resistance while voiding [5]. The urethra is approximately 3-4 cm long and maintains sufficient pressure to prevent urine passage during times of physiological increases such as coughing or physical activities [4].

The urethral lumen is surrounded by several layers of muscle composed of two kinds of muscles, namely, smooth muscle also called the internal urethral sphincter and striated muscle also called the external urethral sphincter.

Both internal and external urethral sphincters play a vital role in maintaining continence. The internal urethral sphincter, smooth muscle beginning at the bladder neck through the proximal urethra, is controlled by the autonomic nervous system.

The external urethral sphincter is muscle fibers from the pubococcygeal muscle of the pelvic floor conformed into a circular manner around the urethra and controlled by the somatic nervous system.

The other striated muscle of the pelvic floor also contributes to the support of the bladder and the urethra as well as continence [2, 7].

Both skeletal and smooth muscles contribute to resting tone while skeletal muscle responds to rises in intra-abdominal pressures [7].

The pelvic floor musculature in females is also important in maintaining continence. The pelvic floor is composed of the levator ani muscles, the supporting ligaments and the endopelvic fascia. These tissues provide support for the urethra by forming a 'hammock' behind the urethra.

During increases in intra-abdominal pressure (such as coughing and sneezing) the urethra is compressed against this hammock, thereby keeping the urethra closed and continent [2, 5].

Micturition, a complex process, is also incorporated in the nervous system including the brain, brain stem, spinal cord, autonomic nervous system, somatic nervous system and neurotransmitters. Urination is composed of two relative discrete phases, namely, the urine storage phase or bladder filling, and the voiding phase or bladder emptying [5].

When the bladder is distended to 150-300 ml during the urine storage phase, stretch receptors in the bladder wall are stimulated by the amount of urine in the bladder and transmit sensory impulses up to the sacral micturition center at the spinal cord. When sufficient urine is present (400-500 ml), the spinal cord transmits autonomic impulses, both sympathetic and parasympathetic, which move down to the detrusor muscle and urethra [5, 8].

In the storage phase, the sympathetic nerves become stimulated, relaxing the detrusor muscle and closing the internal urethral sphincter.

In contrast, parasympathetic nerves become inhibited, hindering detrusor muscle contraction as the somatic pudendal nerve innervation controls the voluntary skeletal muscle of the external urethral sphincter to maintain closure [5]. During the voiding phase, parasympathetic nerves become stimulated and sympathetic nerves become inhibited.

As a result, the contraction of the detrusor muscle and relaxation of the internal urethral sphincter pushes urine flow from the bladder to the urethra and out of the body.

At an inappropriate time and place, the urination is stopped by voluntary contraction of the external urethral sphincter which is under cerebral control [4, 5].

PREVALENCE AND TYPES OF URINARY INCONTINENCE MOST COMMONLY ENCOUNTERED IN PREGNANT WOMEN

The most common type of urinary incontinence (UI) in pregnant women is stress urinary incontinence (SUI). A number of studies have been conducted on the prevalence of SUI during pregnancy. The range of SUI prevalence varies with the prevalence of SUI in the population depending on the use of different study designs, definitions, evaluations, questionnaires and the stage of pregnancy in which data were collected [9-11].

While most population data have focused on European or Western countries, a few studies have determined SUI during pregnancy in Asia, especially in South East Asia. Data from the Norwegian Mother and Child Cohort Study at the Norwegian Institute of Public Health, Wesnes et al. [12] presented questionnaire data about UI obtained from 43,279 pregnant women. They reported that SUI was the most common type of UI during pregnancy, experienced by 31% of nulliparous and 42% of multiparous women. In another study from Norway, Morkved and Bø [13] the researchers investigated the prevalence of SUI during pregnancy and the postpartum period, finding the prevalence of SUI during pregnancy and at 8-weeks after delivery to be 42% and 38%, respectively. In another study from the UK in Europe, Mason et al. [14] found 59% of pregnant women to report SUI during pregnancy, and 10% of the women had daily episodes of incontinence during pregnancy. In Spain, the prevalence of SUI among 596 primigravidae women was 30.3% [15]. In another cross-sectional survey from North-East Scotland, Whitford et al. [16] reported the prevalence of SUI in pregnant women to be 54.3%.

In Germany, Huebner et al. [17] reported data from primigravidae women that UI was estimated at 26.3% and significantly increased during the second half of pregnancy. In Denmark, Viktrup et al. [18] researchers found 4% of primiparous women to have had SUI before pregnancy and 32% during pregnancy, whereas 7% developed postpartum SUI.

The prevalence of UI in Asia is lower compared with Europe. In a large population survey conducted in China among 10,098 Chinese primiparous women, SUI was estimated to be present in 18.6% of pregnant women in late pregnancy [19]. One the prevalence of SUI in Taiwanese primiparous women, 26.7% of the women reported SUI [20].

In another survey, the prevalence of SUI in pregnant women was reported to be 46.1% [21]. In Thailand, the prevalence of UI during pregnancy has been found to be approximately 36.5 % [22].

In South Asia, a survey was conducted in India in which the prevalence of SUI was found to be 19.2% [23]. One study from the Middle East, conducted in Jordan reported the estimated SUI to be approximately 45% of pregnant women [24].

In North America, the highest reported prevalence of SUI is in the United States. According to data from the US, Thomason et al. [25] reported a prevalence of 60% for SUI during pregnancy in continent primiparous women. In another population survey, Raza-Khan et al. [26] reported UI in 70% of nulliparous and 75% of parous women with 32% reporting pure SUI. A high prevalence has also been reported in South America.

In another survey from Brazil, the prevalence of SUI in healthy pregnant Brazilian women was reported to be 46.1% in primigravidae and 54.0 % in multigravidae women [27].

In Australia, Brown et al. [28] reported the prevalence of SUI to be 36.9%, further reporting that SUI was more common during pregnancy than urge incontinence in nulliparous women. Chiarelli and Campbell [29] found 64% of 304 women to report incontinence during pregnancy.

Bø et al. [30] investigated the prevalence of UI in a multi-ethnic population of pregnant women in Norway where all 722 participants were in the first trimester. According to the findings, the lowest prevalence rates of UI at 28 weeks of gestation were 26% for women of African origin. The prevalence of UI in women of Middle Eastern origin was 36%, which was slightly higher than in the women from African origin. Prevalence rates of 40% and 43% were found in women from East Asian origin and South Asian origin, respectively. The highest prevalence was reported at 45% among women from European or North American origin.

Although the prevalence of UI is variant worldwide, most studies have found the prevalence of SUI to generally increase with gestational age [20, 21, 31], peaking during the third trimester, followed by the second and first trimesters [32, 33]. Numerous studies have shown prevalence rates of SUI between 13% and 19% during the first trimester of pregnancy [34, 35] to increase during the second trimester and peak during the third trimester to rates of 19.2% and 37.5%, respectively [20]. According to the study of Wijma et al. [33], the high prevalence of UI during pregnancy was 30% for women at gestational ages of 28-32 weeks, and 35% for pregnant women at gestational ages of 36-38 weeks. Similar findings were reported by Kerrebroeck et al. [36] who showed the prevalence of incontinence to worsen as pregnancy advanced, and reported 17-25% for UI in pregnant women during early pregnancy with an increase to 36-37% in late pregnancy.

According to the above findings in this summary, the number of pregnant women with SUI is variable, prevalence ranges from 18.6% to 75% and SUI prevalence increases with gestational age.

PATHOPHYSIOLOGY OF STRESS URINARY INCONTINENCE DURING PREGNANCY

The pathophysiology of SUI is multifactorial and thought to be related to a general weakening of the pelvic floor muscles and the collagen-dependent tissues involved in pelvic support as a result of pregnancy and parturition [37]. Hilde et al. [38] found continent pregnant women to have significantly higher pelvic floor muscle strength and endurance when compared with pregnant women who have UI.

Under normal conditions, SUI does not occur because of the body's continence mechanism which is dependent on the normal functioning of the lower urinary tract such as the bladder, internal and external sphincter of the urethra.

Furthermore, the pelvic floor muscles have an important role in maintaining the continence mechanism and pelvic organ support [39], thereby indicating that strengthening the pelvic floor muscles may lead to urethral sphincter competence as a result of urethral pressure exceeding bladder pressure and helping to prevent urine leakage with increased intra-abdominal pressure.

Most researchers now accept that the major cause of SUI is multifactorial in which two pathological mechanisms predominate: the bladder neck and urethral hypermobility with intrinsic sphincter deficiency. Most women have elements of both disorders [4, 5, 37]. The weakness of the pelvic floor muscles causes bladder neck and urethral hypermobility, thereby leading to urethral sphincter incompetence [40, 41].

In urethral hypermobility, the basic abnormality is a weakness of pelvic floor muscle support and the urethral support ligaments [5]. Because of this weakness, increases in intra-abdominal pressure result in rotational descent of the bladder neck and proximal urethra.

In intrinsic sphincter deficiency, the urethral sphincteric mechanism that usually contracts to increase sphincteric resistance during increases in intra-abdominal pressure to facilitate sphincter closure and maintains continence is weakened.

Weakness of sphincteric contraction leads to an inability of the urethra to generate sufficient pressure for resistance and increases in intra-abdominal pressure during physical activities such as coughing, sneezing, laughing or moving. The result is SUI [5].

Pregnancy is one of the main risk factors for the development of SUI in young women [42, 43] because pregnancy may be associated with reduced strength of the pelvic floor muscles which can develop into SUI. Interestingly, most women (76%) perceive that they are UI due to weakened pelvic floor muscles [44]. Studies in pregnant women with SUI have found significantly decreased pelvic floor muscle strength in incontinent pregnant women as compared with continent pregnant women [38, 45].

Furthermore, there is a significantly higher prevalence of SUI in pregnant women than in non-pregnant women [43, 46-48].

Pregnancy may be associated with reduced pelvic floor muscle strength which can develop into SUI. However, the exact causes of pregnancy-related SUI remain unclear [49, 50]. During pregnancy, the urogenital system and pelvic floor muscles undergo anatomical and physiological changes [51].

These changes during pregnancy may lead to reduced strength of the pelvic floor muscles and the development of SUI in pregnant women by the aforementioned mechanisms [52].

Pelvic Floor Muscle Trauma Caused by the Uterus and Fetus

The growing uterus and fetal put weight solely on the pelvic floor muscle throughout pregnancy. Pelvic pressure increases as pregnancy progresses. The chronic stress on the pelvic floor muscle results in pelvic floor muscle weakness which plays an important role in the urethral support continent mechanism [41, 47, 53]. As a result of these changes, the strength and supportive sphincteric function of the pelvic floor muscle are jeopardized.

Furthermore, multi-gravidity causes decreased pelvic floor muscle strength at a rate of 22-35% beginning at a gestational age of 20 weeks and lasting until 6 weeks postpartum [40]. Hilde et al. [38] in a cross sectional study of 300 nulliparous women at gestational ages of 18-22 weeks showed continent pregnant women to have significantly higher pelvic floor muscle strength and endurance when compared with incontinent pregnant women ($p=0.003$ and $p=0.01$, respectively).

Bladder neck and urethral hypermobility are a result of the weakness of the pelvic floor muscles supporting the bladder neck and urethra [54]. This prenatal reduction in pelvic floor muscle strength may lead to increased bladder neck and urethral mobility [55, 56] and cause the mobility of the urethrovescicle junction [57]. Urethral mobility is associated with SUI [58].

Wijma et al. [59] found increased bladder neck mobility from early pregnancy onward to near term. Therefore, it is indicated that the mobility of the urethrovescicle junction is associated with an increased risk for SUI during pregnancy and the postpartum period [57].

Jundt et al. [60] found pregnant women with SUI to have more mobile bladder necks than continent pregnant women. Therefore, it is indicated that the mobility of the urethrovescicle junction is associated with an increased risk for SUI during pregnancy and the postpartum period [57].

COLLAGEN CHANGES DURING PREGNANCY

Collagen changes are included in both tensile properties and number. The changes in the tensile properties of the connective tissue contribute to the reduction of functional support of the pelvic floor muscle. While the reduction of total collagen content may result in joint laxity and stretching of the pelvic ligaments [61], the measurement of collagen content and strength is not possible during pregnancy by biopsy.

Although traditional causes such as joint hypermobility and striae have not been predictive for postnatal SUI, bladder neck mobility might be a causal factor [62].

King and Freeman [57] found a 30% incidence of bladder neck mobility in primigravidae women at 19 weeks of pregnancy by using perineal ultrasound, concluding bladder neck mobility to be associated with the development of postnatal SUI at 3 months postpartum.

Several studies have reported a decrease in the total collagen content in women with SUI [55, 63]. Keane et al. [55] showed that nulliparous women with SUI had significantly less collagen content in their tissues compared with continent pregnant women ($p<0.0001$), also concluding that the etiology of SUI in these pregnant women appears to be due to both quantitative and qualitative reductions in collagen.

Hormonal Changes during Pregnancy

The processes affecting pelvic floor function are multifactorial and incompletely understood, but hormone concentrations during and after pregnancy are likely to play a significant role [64]. Hormonal fluctuation can impact not only the genital or gynecological structures but also the lower urinary tract and pelvic floor structure [65]. The following hormonal changes in Relaxin and progesterone during pregnancy may be significant in the development of SUI [66]. Relaxin, a member of the insulin family of the peptide hormone [67], is plays an important role in maintaining urinary continence and can stimulate tissue growth in the lower urinary tract and increase urethral pressure during pregnancy [68].

There is a marked increase in Relaxin concentration during early pregnancy which peaks at a the gestational age of 10-14 weeks and then decreases to approximately half the peak value at the 17th-24th week of pregnancy [69-71] then remains stable until labor and delivery [71]. In contrast to previous studies, Harvey et al. [64] found relaxin tended to be higher at mid-gestational age and fall significantly faster in women with pelvic floor dysfunction (PFD). A decrease in relaxin results in decreased growth of the urethral epithelium which may lead to decreased urethral pressure [49, 61].

Pregnant women with SUI have been found to have lower urethral pressure than continent pregnant women [72]. Harvey et al. [64] found relaxin concentration to decline significantly more rapidly from 24 to 28 weeks of pregnancy in pregnant women with UI. Similarly, Kristiansson et al. [68] found a significant association between low maternal serum relaxin at 18-22 weeks of pregnancy and UI with onset during pregnancy, concluding that lower relaxin concentrations in later pregnancy are, therefore, correlated with a higher prevalence of SUI at the second and third trimesters of pregnancy [68].

Progesterone - During pregnancy, progesterone increases from 24 ng/ml at the 8th week of pregnancy to 150 ng/ml at the 36th week of pregnancy [73]. Increases in progesterone during pregnancy may lead to decreased estrogen receptors. Estrogen plays an important role in the function of the lower urinary tract for maintaining the continence mechanism by encouraging the growth and development of vaginal epithelial cells which make up the thick, healthy layers of the vaginal wall [74], thereby increasing urethral resistance and receptors in the urethral smooth muscle [75].

Hence, increased progesterone may lead to relaxation of the smooth muscle in the urinary system [76], while reducing the tone in the ureter, bladder and urethra which results in SUI during pregnancy [49, 77].

Expansion of the Uterus and Fetal Weight throughout Pregnancy

Two other major factors that influence the incontinence mechanism during pregnancy are the expansion of the uterus and the increment of fetal weight with gestational age, especially during the third trimester.

The aforementioned put direct pressure on the bladder, which may lead to changes in the bladder-neck position and decreased bladder capacity; hence, bladder pressure exceeds the urethral pressure [78], thereby resulting in urine leakage with increased intra-abdominal pressure.

In summary, commonly encountered prenatal physiological changes such as the increasing pressure of the growing uterus and fetal weight on the pelvic floor muscles throughout pregnancy, together with pregnancy-related hormonal changes in progesterone, estrogen and relaxin may lead to reduced strength as well as the supportive and sphincteric function of the pelvic floor muscles. The weakness of the pelvic floor muscles causes mobility of the bladder neck and urethra, thereby leading to urethral sphincter incompetence or intrinsic sphincter deficiency.

As a result, urethral sphincter incompetence may lead to urethral pressure that is less than bladder pressure and intra-abdominal pressure. Hence, when intra-abdominal pressure increases during physical activities such as coughing, sneezing, laughing or moving, the pressure inside the bladder becomes greater than the urethral closure pressure and the urethral sphincter is not strong enough to close the urethra; the consequence is SUI [52].

Factors Increasing the Risk of Developing Stress Urinary Incontinence among Pregnant Women

The following section discusses the risk factors for the development of SUI in pregnant women. Understanding of this topic can be useful for health professionals in informing and counseling pregnant women to prevent and reduce the risk factors contributing to the development of SUI during pregnancy and the postpartum period.

Multiple factors have been found to be associated with the development of SUI during pregnancy, including the following.

1. Age

Age: SUI during pregnancy is associated with advanced maternal age [12]. Zhu et al. [19] reported that the risk of SUI incidence increases with maternal age (OR 1.041, 95%CI 1.027- 1.055). These findings are supported by Hvidman et al. [79] who found pregnant women aged 30 years and older to be at significantly greater risk for SUI than younger women (OR=1.4). This finding is significant evidence emphasizing the role of maternal age at the time of first pregnancy as an independent risk factor for the occurrence of SUI [80]. Groutz et al. [81] reported that older maternal age of over 30 years at first birth was also significant risk factor for persistent and long-term UI. This finding was also supported by Glazener et al. [82] who found the maternal age to be an independent risk factor on the new onset of UI with increased risk for older women at 35 years and over. Older age at first delivery may be a risk factor for pelvic floor trauma [83] in older pregnant women because advanced maternal age leads to loss of nerve function and urethral closure pressure [84], as well as decreases in the total number of striated muscle fibers of the urethral sphincter at a rate of 2% a year [85, 86]. Furthermore, older maternal age before the first pregnancy is a contributing factor affecting the degree of injury to the pelvic floor muscle [87]. Trowbridge et al. [88] conducted a cohort study to evaluate the effects of aging on urethral support, urethral function and levator function in 82 nulliparous women. According to the findings, increasing age was associated with decreasing maximal urethral closure pressure ($r=-0.758$, $P<.001$); however, pelvic organ support, urethral support and levator function have not been found to change with increasing age.

In contrast, few studies show the association between women with younger age and SUI. Hojberg et al. [46] reported that younger pregnant women aged between 15 to 24 years had a significantly higher risk for SUI than those aged between 25 to 29 years (OR=1.5; 95% CI 1.0-2.4).

Furthermore, Lewicky-Gaupp et al. [89] determined the prevalence of UI during pregnancy in adolescent African-American women, finding a high prevalence of SUI in adolescent pregnant women during the third trimester at 43%.

2. Parity

Parity: The number of previous pregnancies and deliveries is significantly higher in incontinent pregnant women than continent pregnant women [27].

This finding was supported by Wesnes et al. [12] who investigated the associated risk factors for UI during pregnancy among 43,279 pregnant women, finding parity to be a strong and significant risk factor for incontinence in adjusted analyses both before pregnancy (odds ratio [OR] 2.5, 95% confidence interval [CI] 2.4-2.7 for primiparous and OR 3.3, 95% CI 3.1-3.5 for multiparous women) and during pregnancy (ORs 2.0, 95% CI 1.9-2.1 and 2.1, 95% CI 2.0-2.2, respectively). Arrue et al. [90] suggested the mechanism causing the association between parity and SUI might be related to the hormonal changes occurring during gestation. Primiparae who deliver vaginally are also at a significantly higher risk for SUI than nulliparae.

Furthermore, multiparous women are associated with greater risk for SUI than primiparae [46, 91].

A study by Marshall et al. [92] reported a high reverse association in percentage of UI and number of parity at 68% of multiparous women who had given birth five times or more as compared to 66% in multiparous women who had given birth 2-4 times and 55.0% for primigravidae.

3. Mode of Delivery

Mode of Delivery: Vaginal delivery is associated with pelvic floor dysfunction and reduced urethral closure pressure. Furthermore, bladder neck mobility is increased significantly after all vaginal births [93]. These changes are caused by traction or stretching of the pudendal nerve fibers that supply the pelvic floor muscle [80, 94-96]. Tunn et al. [97] suggested that vaginal childbirth results in neuromuscular and ischemic damage in the bladder outlet and urethra, thereby increasing the risk for SUI.

The damage to pelvic floor musculature, fascial support and nerve supply usually occurs during the second stage of labor when the mother pushes and the fetal head distends and stretches the pelvic floor [80].

Numerous studies have reported the impact of the mode of delivery on the development of UI in women, comparing the effects of caesarean section and vaginal delivery. In the largest study carried out in an Italian population, Torrisi et al. [98] confirmed that vaginal delivery is a strong important risk factors for the development of UI (OR 3.3, CI 2.0-5.3, p<.001).

In a population-based cohort study by Leijonhufvud et al. [99], the researchers estimated the risk of SUI related to vaginal birth or cesarean delivery in 60,122 women with vaginal delivery and 30,880 women with cesarean delivery.

According to the findings, there was a significantly increased risk for SUI later in life among the women who had delivered only by vaginal childbirth compared to those having only cesarean delivery.

Primiparae who deliver vaginally are also at significantly higher risk for SUI than nulliparae (OR 5.9; 95% CI 4.1-8.3). Furthermore, multiparous women are associated with greater risk for SUI than primiparae [46, 91].

A study by Marshall et al. [92] reported a high percentage of UI of approximately 68% in multiparous women who had given birth five times or more as compared to 66% in multiparous women who had given birth 2-4 times and 55.0% for primigravidae.

In addition, Yang et al. [100] found an increase in the prevalence of SUI after forceps delivery compared to vaginal delivery, assessing 1,889 primiparous postpartum women and finding SUI prevalence to be related to vaginal delivery (OR 5.42, 95% CI 2.60-11.32, $p=0.000$) and forceps delivery (OR 7.0, 95% CI 2.40-20.41, $p=0.000$). They concluded that vaginal delivery had a risk impact on UI in postpartum women, especially in cases involving forceps delivery. Goldberg et al. [101] reported that women delivering vaginally demonstrated a significantly higher rate of SUI than women who deliver by cesarean section (OR 2.28, CI 1.14-4.55, $p<0.019$). In contrast, Arrue et al. [90] found no statistically significant association between the mode of vaginal delivery and SUI 6 months after delivery.

UI is commonly found in women with instrumental compared to spontaneous vaginal delivery (36% and 34%, respectively), and lowest in women with elective cesarean section (13%) [102]. These results are consistent with the study of Arya et al. [103] who found forceps delivery to be associated with higher risk for SUI compared with spontaneous vaginal delivery. The increased incidence of SUI associated with forceps delivery may be related to the accelerated descent of the fetal head by forceps extraction as compared to normal labor. Forceps delivery causes more stretching which damages the nerves and connective tissue of the pelvic floor [104].

Cesarean section could have a protective role in postpartum SUI in comparison with vaginal delivery [105, 106]. Women with cesarean section are at lower risk for postpartum SUI than those with vaginal delivery [107]. This finding is supported by Boyles et al. [108] who reported that cesarean section reduced the risk of postpartum SUI and found pregnant women who had had vaginal deliveries to be more likely to have SUI than women who had had cesarean deliveries (odds ratio of 4.96 [95% confidence interval 3.82-6.44], P<.001). Fritel et al. [109] reported cesarean delivery to be associated with lower rates of SUI than vaginal delivery.

However, cesarean section is not associated with a major reduction of UI [110], which concurs with the findings of Chou et al. [111] who reported cesarean section to not prevent SUI in primiparous mothers at 1 year postpartum.

4. Obesity, High Body Mass Index (BMI) and High Weight Gain during Pregnancy

Obesity, high body mass index (BMI) and high weight gain during pregnancy: Another risk factor for SUI during pregnancy is obesity or high body mass index (BMI) [112]. Increased body mass index (BMI) before pregnancy has been found to be associated with an increased risk for developing stress incontinence and appears to be linear in that the higher the BMI, the greater the risk of developing incontinence [113]. Several studies have shown the association between the obesity and SUI. Zhu et al. [19] reported the risk of SUI to increase with increasing prenatal BMI (OR=1.037). Furthermore, the physiological weight gain during pregnancy may lead to increased pressure on the PFM and bladder which may result in greater urethral mobility [114, 115]. Moreover, obesity may impair blood flow and nerve innervation to the bladder and urethra [116] with increased BMI correlated with increased intra-abdominal pressure during urodynamic assessments and increased the risk of SUI later in life [115, 117]. Glazener et al. [82] found women with UI first occurring during pregnancy to be associated with higher BMI > 25 (OR 1.68, 95%CI 1.12-2.43). In the study of Hojberg et al. [46] it was reported that pregnant women with pre-pregnancy BMI of more than 30 kg/m^2 and 35 kg/m^2 were at significantly higher risk for SUI than those with a normal pre-pregnancy BMI (OR=1.7; 95% CI 0.9-3.2 and OR=2.5; 95% CI 1.0-6.0, respectively).

Similarly, Hvidman et al. [79] found pregnant women with a pre-pregnancy BMI of more than 30 kg/m^2 to be associated with a high rate of SUI (OR=2.2). Liang et al. [20] reported that women with a pre-pregnancy BMI of more than 30 kg/m^2 to be at increased risk for developing SUI during pregnancy. Brown et al. [28] reported that pregnant women with a BMI 30 kg/m^2 or more were at increased risk for developing de novo UI during pregnancy (AdjOR=1.5, 95% CI 1.0-2.3). Diez-Itza et al. [15] found the women at term pregnancy with at term body weight of 75 kg or more to have more than doubled the risk for SUI.

These findings are similar to the study of Arrue et al. [90] who reported continent primigravida women who had higher weight gain in pregnancy to have increased the risk for SUI after delivery.

5. Smoking

Smoking - Smoking is also a contributing risk factor for SUI [118, 119]. Carbon monoxide in cigarettes impairs oxygen transported to bodily tissues and results in muscle atrophy. The pelvic floor muscle are also affected. Chronic and frequent coughing exerting significant pressure to the pelvic floor muscle may lead to damaging innervation to the pelvic floor muscle and aggravated SUI. Not only carbon monoxide, but also the nicotine have a stimulating effect on the detrusor muscle. The chronic nicotinic detrusor muscle stimulation accompanied by increased intra-abdominal pressure contributes to urine leakage [120].

Hojberg et al. [46] reported pregnant women who smoke to be at a significantly higher risk for SUI during pregnancy compared to non-smoking pregnant women (OR 1.4; 95% CI 1.1-1.9). Martins et al. [27] reported that 12.4% of Brazilian women smoked during pregnancy, and found significant association between UI and smoking among incontinent pregnant women (p=0.010). Similarly, Liang et al. [20] found 6.8% of pregnant women who reported smoking in pregnancy, an incident associated with urge UI, but found no association with SUI.

6. Constipation

Constipation: During pregnancy, constipation is a common symptom caused by reduced intestinal movement, the progesterone effect, and the weight of the expanding uterus that presses against the bowel and peristalsis. These changes may result in hard and dry stool causing pelvic floor muscle damage [121]. Marshall et al. [92] found a high percentage of constipation at approximately 37% of pregnant women. Constipation most frequently occurs during the third trimester of pregnancy [92, 122, 123]. Constipation may be associated as risk for SUI as the hard stool presses the urethra, affecting nerve innervation and blood flow to the urethral sphincter and potentially resulting in sphincteric deficiency [124]. In addition, constipation adds significant pressure to the bladder and urethra during defecation, which may also lead to UI.

Amselem et al. [125] found constipation to be identified in 31% (19/61) of women with pelvic floor damage. In women without pelvic floor damage, constipation was present in 16% (83/535).

These results indicated constipation to be as important as obstetric trauma in the development of PFM damage.

Treatment of constipation might significantly reduce the prevalence of this distressing problem. Martins et al. [27] found 67.5% (168/249) of Brazilian pregnant women with constipation (bowel movements less than 3 times per week) to have UI during pregnancy (p=0.02), further reporting the risk factor associated with UI during pregnancy to be constipation.

Zhu et al. [19] reported that women with a history of constipation were more likely to develop SUI in late pregnancy (OR=1.218) and the difficult defecation was a risk factor for the development of UI during late pregnancy to 6 weeks postpartum (OR=1.629).

7. Pre-Pregnancy Stress Urinary Incontinence

Pre-pregnancy stress urinary incontinence: Urine leakage prior the current pregnancy or in previous pregnancies could be a sign of poor quality of the connective tissue of the pelvic floor muscle [126] and may reduce fascia tensile strength during pregnancy more than in previously continent women [127]. The weakness of the pelvic floor muscle resulting in the loss of the supportive mechanism of the urethra and bladder neck further contributes to the risk for SUI [126].

Pre-pregnancy SUI indicates the risk factor for developing UI during pregnancy and postpartum. Hvidman et al. [79] reported that previously incontinent pregnant women had significantly higher risk for SUI in pregnancy than previously continent pregnant women (OR 10.6).

According to the study of Stainton et al. [128], women who experience urine leakage prior to pregnancy are at risk and contribute to postnatal UI (P = 0.02). These findings were supported by Brown et al. [28] who examined the association between pre-pregnancy UI and UI during pregnancy in 1,507 nulliparous women.

According to the findings, the strongest predictor of incidence of UI during pregnancy was occasional pre-pregnancy urine leakage (AdjOR 3.6, 95% CI 2.8-4.7).

8. History of Gestational Diabetes Mellitus (hGDM)

History of gestational diabetes mellitus (hGDM) The direct association between women with hGDM and SUI is undetermined. Few studies have reported women with hGDM to have a high prevalence of UI because of their higher BMI, obesity and macrosomia of infants [129, 130]. However, the exact mechanism remains unclear and excess weight gain during pregnancy may exert pressure on the pelvic floor muscle, which increases pressure on bladder and urethral mobility, thereby leading to UI [131].

In a cross-sectional survey, Kim et al. [132] examined the prevalence of SUI among women with hGDM, surveying 228 women with hGDM over the past 5 years after delivery and finding 49% of women with hGDM to report weekly or more frequent incontinence during pregnancy; 50% of the women reported postpartum SUI. Therefore, the high prevalence of obesity may have contributed to the high prevalence of SUI during pregnancy and after delivery among the participants. The aformentioned study found obesity in 42% of women during pregnancy and 46% after delivery.

However, there was no clear association between BMI and SUI. Thus, the researchers concluded that SUI was common among women with hGDM.

Only one study found an association between GDM and SUI during the postpartum period. Chuang et al. [133] conducted a survey of 6,653 pregnant women with GDM to determine whether GDM is an independent risk factor for SUI postpartum. According to the findings, pregnant women with GDM tend toward exhibiting more severe SUI symptoms for up 2 years postpartum compared with women without GDM (OR 1.97, 95% CI 1.56–2.51).

Therefore, the researchers concluded that GDM was found to be an independent risk factor for UI postpartum and significantly associated with impact on QOL [133].

9. Alcohol and Caffeine Consumption

Alcohol and Caffeine Consumption: Few studies examined the association between alcohol intake and UI. Only one study reported an associated between alcohol consumption and SUI in pregnancy. Zhu et al. [19] reported that primiparous women who drank alcohol had a higher risk factor for developing SUI in late pregnancy than those who did not (OR 1.221).

Another study investigated the association between alcohol consumption and UI among non-pregnant women.

Among 298 eligible middle-aged and older Japanese women, Lee and Hirayama [134], found, 82 women (27.5%) to experience urine leakage. The prevalence of alcohol drinking and mean ethanol intake was slightly higher among the incontinent women (39%; 7.1, SD 24.1 g/day) than others without the condition (35.6%; 4.3, SD 10.7 g/day). However, the association between alcohol consumption and UI is less clear [134].

Nevertheless, the study did find a strong association between daily coffee consumption and UI [135]. These findings were confirmed by Martins et al. [27] who found the risk factors associated with UI during pregnancy to include smoking, constipation and coffee consumption, reporting that pregnant women who consumed two or more cups of coffee a day were 1.7 times more likely to report UI (p=0.008). For the non-pregnant population, Gleason et al. [136] investigated the associations between caffeine consumption and severity of UI in 4,309 nulliparous women in the US, finding the prevalence of any UI to be 41.0 % with SUI as the most common type (36.6 %). After adjusting for multiple factors, caffeine intake in the highest quartile was associated with any UI. Type of UI (stress, urgency, mixed) was not associated with caffeine intake. Hence, the researchers concluded that high caffeine intake ≥204 mg/day was associated with any type of UI.

With regard to the aforementioned findings, Sangsawang and Sangsawang [52] found the prevalence of SUI among pregnant women to be reported at rates of 18.6% to 75%, meaning that the remaining approximate 25% of pregnant women do not develop SUI during pregnancy.

Therefore, the physiological changes during pregnancy do not lead to SUI in every pregnant woman [137]. Rather, SUI during pregnancy is associated with a lack of pelvic floor muscle strength. Therefore, any factors causing weakening of pelvic floor muscle strength are likely to be causal factors for SUI during pregnancy. Several factors may decrease the strength of pelvic floor muscle in addition to pregnancy itself [137].

These risk factors include the age, obesity, smoking, constipation, pre-pregnancy SUI and gestational diabetes mellitus in which no associations have been found among the risk factors [137]. This means that each risk factor is independent and will independently result in SUI. Therefore, pregnant women do not need to have all of the risk factors in order to develop SUI during pregnancy. Pregnant women may have only one or a combination of multiple risk factors to cause SUI and various risk factors will result in a lack of pelvic floor muscle strength with the possibility of developing SUI [137].

In summary, the mechanisms of the risk factors involved in developing SUI during pregnancy include the following three domains: 1) increased intra-abdominal pressure; 2) increased pressure to the bladder, urethra and pelvic floor muscle and 3) impaired blood flow, oxygen transportation and innervation to the bladder, urethra and pelvic floor muscle [137]. These factors have the effect of weakening the pelvic floor muscle, the major supportive of continence mechanism, and leading to pelvic floor and urethral dysfunction with loss of uretharal closure pressure [137].

In addition, obesity, smoking, and constipation are independent risk factors that cause SUI during pregnancy. These factors can be avoided and prevented [137] with behavioral modification during pregnancy. Effective means of preventing SUI during pregnancy are aimed at strengthening the pelvic floor muscle and avoiding the risks of weakening pelvic floor muscle strength [137].

Although some are less clear, many modifiable and non-modifiable risk factors have been identified as risks contributing to the effects of the major supportive mechanism of the bladder and PFM [137]. Nevertheless, non-modifiable, genetic and obstetric risk factors such as age, pre-pregnancy SUI and GDM have an important role in SUI development.

Factors such as obesity, smoking and constipation are modifiable risk factors. Avoiding modifiable risk factors might reduce the risk for development of SUI in pregnant women. Prevention of SUI during pregnancy may also reduce the incidence of SUI during the postpartum period [137].

Investigation and Assessment of Stress Urinary Incontinence

A variety of investigations are available for diagnosing SUI and can be categorized as history, physical examination, urinalysis, post-void residual urine volume, urodynamic studies and ultrasound [138, 139].

1. History

History is the primary essential factor for the evaluation of women with SUI. History can usually reveal the type, severity and difficulty of incontinence. Women should be queried about urological history, including voiding patterns, frequency and characteristics of urine leakage, as well as related symptoms such as urgency, frequency, nocturia and dysuria.

Furthermore, the evaluator must query patients about obstetric history and modes of delivery, gynecological history, smoking history, history of alcohol and caffeine consumption, history of previous pelvic surgery or radiotherapy that may have damaged the pelvic nerve supply to the pelvic floor muscles and urethra. History of chronic diseases such as diabetes, chronic urinary tract infection and bowel history such as symptoms of constipation, diarrhea, diet and fluid intake as well as history of medications prescribed and taken should also be determined.

The degree of difficulty or inconvenience from symptoms is important when planning treatment. In particular, the predominant problem should be defined in women with mixed symptoms. Useful tools are validated condition-specific symptom and quality of life questionnaires such as the King's Health Questionnaire and the combined ICIQ UI SF.

The history alone can be relatively conclusive of the final urodynamic diagnosis of SUI in which the isolated symptoms of SUI show a positive predictive value of 79% for urodynamic SUI.

2. Physical Examination

Physical examination can help to exclude concomitant pathology, for example pelvic organ prolapse and pelvic mass. SUI can also be identified by a cough stress test. Physical examination should begin by observing the patient as she enters the room in an attempt to detect signs of a neurological condition. The patient may be examined while she is standing, sitting or in the lithotomy position [140]. The examination should include the following:

2.1. Neurologic examination: The neurologic examination is divided into four parts including mental status, sensory function, motor function and deep tendon reflexes. The neurologic examination should begin by observing the patient as she enters the room to assess mobility.

Mental status can be evaluated by observing the patient’s level of alertness, orientation, speech patterns and memory. Inspect the spinal curvature from posterior and lateral positions for spinal surgical incisions. Sensory function and motor function can be evaluated by twelve pairs of cranial nerves and thirty-one pairs of spinal nerves.

Assessment of neurologic reflexes can be made through both deep tendon reflex and superficial reflex.

These observations are essential because neurologic dysfunctions may contribute to urinary incontinence.

2.2. Abdominal examination: Abdominal examination should begin with inspection of the condition of the skin and surgical incisions followed by palpation or percussion to assess abnormal masses or tumors. For example, a full bladder may indicate that urine remains in the bladder after the patient's voiding; this can contribute to UI.

2.3. Vaginal examination: Vaginal examination should begin with inspection of the perineal skin as evidence of UI may be found to induce irritant dermatitis. The vaginal mucosa is inspected for evidence of hypoestrogenic atrophy and pelvic organ prolapse such as cystocele, uterine prolapse and vaginal vault prolapse. The palpation can evaluate pelvic masses or tumors putting pressure or irritation on the bladder and voluntary pelvic floor contraction.

The tone and strength of the pelvic floor muscles should be assessed. This can be done by inspection (drawing up of the anus, lifting of the posterior wall of the vagina and narrowing of the vaginal introitus), digital palpation (e.g. the Oxford score) or more advanced techniques such as perineometry and electromyography.

2.4. Stress test: A stress test is performed to examine and assess the urine leakage and can be started when the patient's bladder is full; if the bladder is not already full, a catheter will be necessary and approximately 300 cc. of a water will be inserted into the bladder through the catheter.

The patient may be asked to assume a standing position as a brown piece of paper is lightly placed beneath her perineum and she deeply coughs a few times. The stress test will then be examined for evidence of moisture caused by urine leakage which may indicate SUI.

2.5. Bonney test: The Bonney test is performed to assess after a stress test verifies that urine is lost with the patient's cough or performance of Valsalva's maneuver. The examiner elevates the bladder neck with a finger inserted into the vagina while the patient coughs again. If the urine leakage is stopped when a finger is inserted into the vagina to elevate the bladder neck, the test is considered positive and urethral hypermobility may be indicated. Surgical therapy by elevation of the bladder neck can cure or relieve this condition. It is cautioned, however, that the finger performing the Bonney test must be carefully inserted to avoid directly compressing the urethra and reflecting a false positive.

2.6. Q-tip test: The Q-tip test helps to identify the degree of urethral hypermobility. The patient may be asked to lie in a supine position as the mestus of the urethra is cleaned and a lubricated cotton bud (Q-tip) is inserted into the urethra then pulled back until some resistance is encountered at the urethrovescical junction. The patient is then asked to perform Valsalva's maneuver or cough while the angle of Q-tip is observed.

A change in the Q-tip angle of more than 30° with Valsalva's maneuver indicates mobility of the bladder neck and urethra.

3. Urinalysis

Urinalysis is mandatory as a screening tool for haematuria, glycosuria, pyuria and bacteriuria as indicators of underlying pathology. The urinalysis can detect nitrite, leucocytes, glucose and protein in screening methods for urinary tract infection which is the most common cause of transient conditions possibly contributing to UI because infection can stimulate exotoxin of bacteria for detrusor muscle activity, decrease periurethral muscle tone and urethral pressure potentially developing into SUI in women.

Hematuria may indicate a urethral system tumor and additional evaluation to exclude this condition is necessary before urinary incontinence treatment begins. Proteinuria can be a sign of renal disease. Glycosuria can be a sign of diabetes mellitus, a disease that can cause UI via several mechanisms, such as neuropathy, polyuria and recurrent UTI.

4. Post-Void Residual Urine Volume

Post-void residual urine volume should be estimated, especially in patients with symptoms of voiding difficulty and incomplete bladder emptying. Post-void residual urine volume is performed to assess any urine remaining in the bladder after the patient has attempted to completely empty her bladder. Measurement may be performed by catheterization in which the catheter is inserted into the urethra to drain the remaining urine or ultrasonography wherein ultrasound waves are used to produce shadow-like images when directed at the bladder. These images can detect the amount of residual urine in the bladder. A residual urine volume of less than 50 ml is considered as normal whereas more than 100 ml may indicate abnormality.

5. Urodynamic Studies

Urodynamic studies are not required as part of the initial management of incontinence unless there is voiding dysfunction and high post-void residual volumes or the incontinence is so severe that surgery is indicated as first-line treatment [139]. Urodynamic studies are performed to assess bladder filling and urethral function and can investigate the causes of SUI that are not related to bladder dysfunction. Urodynamic assessment usually includes urinary flow study, bladder and perineal ultrasound, cystometry and urethral pressure profiles. For example, cystometry assesses bladder filling, storage and pressure to diagnose detrusor instability. Urethral pressure profiles measure maximal urethral pressure to determine the measure of maximal urethral pressure in which less than 20 cm H_2O is considered intrinsic sphincter deficiency.

6. Ultrasound

Ultrasound - Similarly, renal and pelvic ultrasound examinations in the initial stage of management can be limited to those patients with suspected pathology. Imaging, however, plays an important role in specialized management.

Impact of Urinary Incontinence on Quality of Life in Pregnant Women

Quality of life (QOL) is an abstract and highly subjective concept as individual assessment of the quality of life can be influenced by personal and cultural values, beliefs, self-concept, goals, age and life expectancy, all of which differ from person to person.

Furthermore, the concept is affected by a broad spectrum of human experiences including disease, interpersonal relationships and social support. Quality of life is usually measured by using structured questionnaires which can be completed by the women or by a structured interview [141].

Structured questionnaires and interviews to assess quality of life with regard to UI contain a varied number of domains that gather information focused on particular aspects of health and covering four domains including physical activity, travel, social relationships and emotional health [142].

Urinary incontinence is common in women and can have a substantial impact on individual quality of life [143]. Although UI is not a life-threatening disorder, it is a condition that causes considerable distress in the form of physical discomfort, economic burden, shame and loss of self-confidence, not to mention sexual function, thereby diminishing quality of life [144, 145].

However, quality of life has been found to be correlated with the severity of UI and women who have UI have reported significant reductions in quality of life [146]. Urinary incontinence affects the quality of life of pregnant women in four domains including physical activity, travel, social relationships and emotional health. More specifically, several pregnant women have responded that urinary incontinence restricts lifestyles, inhibits daily activities, interferes with relationships and results in a loss of self-confidence.

Furthermore, feelings of embarrassment, worry, depression and anxiety have all been found to be associated with the occurrence of urinary incontinence.

Mascarenhas et al. [147] reported that urinary incontinence negatively affects social relationships and particularly interferes with sexual relationships. According to Dolan et al. [148] urinary incontinence has been found to impinge on sexual relationships.

Urinary incontinence has a greater impact on the quality of life of approximately 54.3% pregnant women [148]. Pregnant women with UI have statistically significant lower qualities of life during pregnancy than those without UI [147]. Furthermore, the quality of life of incontinent pregnant women worsens with increasing gestational age to term [149]. This is in correlation with the severity of UI during pregnancy which also increases with gestational age to term.

However, most pregnant women who have UI report a minimal impact on their quality of life [148, 149], therefore, the quality of life of pregnant women has been found to be mildly affected by UI [143]. Dolan et al. [148] found 75.8% of the women to report their quality of life as being affected 'a little' during the antenatal period, while 87.5% said they were affected during the postpartum period. Kocaoz et al. [143] found the quality of life of 70.8% of women experiencing UI to be negatively affected; however, the bothersome effects remained mostly at the mild or moderate level, possibly because the UI symptoms reported by the women were not severe [150] and the women considered the UI a temporary inconvenience [143].

Furthermore, pregnant women tend to consider SUI a common discomfort with symptoms usually occurring during pregnancy due to anatomical, hormonal and mechanical changes and as a sequel of childbirth during the postnatal period [151].

In addition to the impact on the quality of life during pregnancy, another important impact of SUI is identified in an increased risk for permanent incontinence during the postpartum period and later in life [9, 18, 39, 49, 57, 112, 152].

Antenatal SUI is also a well-reported risk factor for long-term SUI. However, although the majority of pregnant women with SUI generally improve after childbirth, not all are as fortunate. Therefore, women who develop SUI during pregnancy without a remission of three months after delivery appear to be a high-risk group for long-term incontinence [62].

Many studies have reported that women who have UI during pregnancy are a more significant predictor of postpartum UI than continent pregnant women. For example, Viktrup et al. [18] and Hvidman et al. [153] found women with urinary leakage during pregnancy to be at significantly greater risk for postpartum UI than those with continence (OR 3.5, $p < 0.000$ and OR 8.5, respectively).

These findings are similar to the findings of Dimpl et al. [154] who reported a strong association between urinary incontinence during pregnancy and the risk of postpartum UI (OR 3.5, $p<0.05$). Foldspang et al. [155] found approximately 66% of women with urinary leakage during pregnancy to report a higher percentage of postpartum UI compared to continent women. Torrisi et al. [98] reported that women who have a new onset of SUI during pregnancy are an independent predictor for persistent UI during the early postpartum period (OR 4.6, 95% CI 3.1-6.8, $P<.001$). Wesnes et al. [102] found an odds ratio of 3.5 for UI at 6 months postpartum among women who were incontinent during pregnancy as opposed to women who were continent during pregnancy.

Moreover, Fritel et al. [126] found women with SUI during their first pregnancy to be at significantly greater risk for SUI for four years after their first delivery (OR 2.5; 95% CI 1.3-4.8). According to the findings of the study of Viktrup and Lose [10], urinary leakage during first pregnancies significantly increases the risk of SUI over the next five years following delivery (OR 3.8; 95% CI 1.9-7.5). Nevertheless, the impact of SUI among women varies with differing individual perceptions, duration and severity of SUI.

Hermansen et al. [44] found half of a group of postnatal women to report small amounts of urine leakage and leakage related to physical activity, coughing or sneezing to indicate that they were moderately or greatly bothered by the leakage. Furthermore, some women living with UI were affected in terms of willingness to go to places where they were unsure about the availability of toilets (27%) and the way they dressed (31%).

Some women reported diminished ability to have sexual relations (23%) and reduced involvement in physical and recreational activities (23%). Moreover, the women were found to associate UI with feelings of frustration (25%) and embarrassment (25%).

STRESS URINARY INCONTINENCE AND SEVERITY ASSESSMENT

Assessment of the severity of SUI usually considers the volume of urine loss, frequency or number of episodes of urine leakage and perceived severity of SUI. Hence, this assessment can be divided into two dimensions including objective and subjective dimensions.

1. Objective Assessment

Objective assessment is a concrete measurement that can evaluated by, for example, the frequency or number of weekly urine leakage episodes [61, 156], the number of sanitary pads used per day [148, 157] or the volume of urine leakage [158, 159]. The overall severity of SUI can generally be categorized into three levels, i.e. mild, moderate and severe. Patients are asked about the number of weekly urine leakage episodes.

Reports of urine leakage episodes occurring approximately once per week, 2-6 times per week or 7 times and more per week are defined as mild, moderate or severe, respectively [57, 148. 159].

The volume of urine leakage is assessed by asking patients about the amount of urine lost wherein reports of less than ½ teaspoon per day are defined as mild and reports of more than a quarter of a cup per day are defined as severe; reports falling between mild and severe are defined as mild [160].

Moreover, the volume of urine leakage can be assessed and estimated by the amount of moisture in underwear after urine loss. This assessment can be categorized into four levels such as no leakage, dampness, wetness or soaking [161].

2. Subjective Assessment

Subjective assessment is a woman's perception of the severity or problems associated with SUI. The visual analogue scale (VAS) is a generally accepted measurement instrument for evaluating the impact of disease on the quality of life and has also been used in evaluating the impact of SUI on quality of life [162, 163]. An effective instrument with high sensitivity as well as reliability and validity, the visual analogue scale is convenient and easy to use.

For example, the reliability of the VAS has been tested using Spearman's rank correlation coefficient in which the score between test-retest was .85 which proved to be valid and responsive in measuring for the severity of urinary incontinence in women [164]. The VAS consists of a 10 cm line, which may be either horizontal or vertical. For a horizontal line, scores range from "0" at the left end, which usually indicates "no problem at all" to 10 at the right end, which represents "can't think of anything worse [157] as shown below:

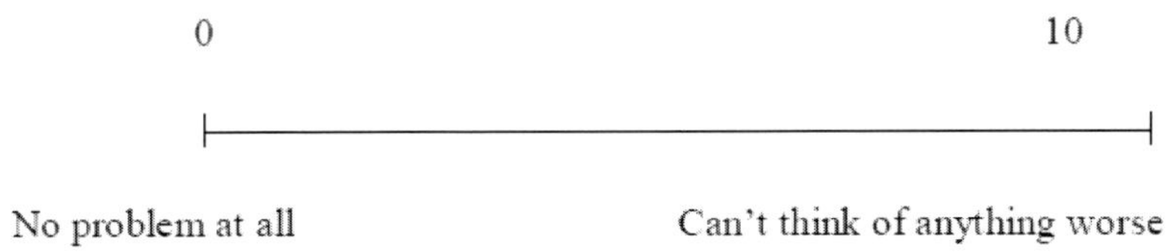

Figure 1. Horizontal Visual Analogue Scale.

To assess the severity of SUI with a visual analogue scale, the patient is asked to place a mark on the line to reflect the level of perceived severity of SUI. To score the results, a ruler is placed along the line and the distance from the patient's mark is measured from the left end and reported in centimeters or millimeters. The objectively assessed impact of UI on the quality of life is not, however, directly related to the subjectively measured degree of UI. Hence, the severity of SUI is assessed with respect to both objective and subjective assessment dimensions. Some women, for example, may positively perceive the severity of SUI as no particular disturbance, even though they experience higher frequency and volume of urine leakage. Therefore, a person's inappropriate perception of severity of SUI may be in conflict with objectively measured assessments [163]. Although UI is not life threatening, it affects the quality of life and inhibits the daily activities of women. Hence, appropriate therapy capable of either curing or alleviating SUI can enhance quality of life.

PART II: PELVIC FLOOR MUSCLE EXERCISE TO PREVENT AND TREAT STRESS URINARY INCONTINENCE DURING PREGNANCY

Current findings indicate that SUI in female and elderly adults can be cured by many treatments with conservative treatment including pelvic floor muscles exercises (PFME), lifestyle and behavioural therapy, and hormonal and pharmacological therapy and surgical treatments such as tension-free vaginal taping (TVT), transvaginal obturator tape (TOT) and retropubic colposuspension [31, 165].

However, conservative therapy is considered the first-line of therapy or treatment for SUI because it not only has few adverse effects but is also effective in controlling urine leakage associated with pelvic floor muscle dysfunction. This method, however, requires a strong commitment from both patients and health care professionals in order to result in successful treatment [152].

Conservative therapy by PFME is the first treatment option [31] for pregnant women with SUI during pregnancy and the postpartum period. Other treatments, whether medical or surgical, must not be proposed as the first intention during pregnancy or the immediate postpartum period [31]. Groenen et al. [166] recommended that pregnant women who had SUI and still wanted to conceive or women who wanted to become pregnant after previous mid-urethral sling surgery wait for completion of all childbearing before any incontinence surgery. If a woman becomes pregnant after mid-urethral sling surgery, no specific treatments need to be taken as long as she remains continent during pregnancy. If she develops SUI again, there is no surgical treatment for SUI during pregnancy and the most appropriate treatment option is to institute conservative treatment [166].

In summary, conservative therapy is generally considered the first-line of treatment for SUI because it is the least invasive treatment and incurs the lowest risk for adverse effects. PFME is the first-line treatment before consideration of other treatments [167] and PFME is an effective treatment for SUI during pregnancy [42, 113, 161] because PFME is a safe, complication-free, inexpensive treatment requiring no instruments and can be done anywhere and anytime [168, 169]. Moreover, following clear instructions, PFME can be performed by women on a regular basis [170].

PELVIC FLOOR MUSCLES EXERCISE (PFME)

The Cochrane review concluded that pregnant women without prior UI who practice intensive antenatal PFME are 56% less likely to report UI in late pregnancy and 30% less like during 6 months postpartum than women who do not practice PFME. Hence, the indication is that antenatal PFME can prevent and treat UI during late pregnancy and the postpartum period [171].

PFME is the most commonly recommended conservative therapy for women with SUI, but it is also sometimes recommended for mixed UI, and less commonly in urgency UI [172].

Pelvic floor muscles or Kegel exercises by alternately contracting and relaxing the pelvic floor muscles are the most commonly recommended conservative therapy for women with SUI.

PFME is used to improve the strength and endurance of the pelvic floor and periurethral muscles; herefore, a strong pelvic floor muscle contraction will clamp the urethra, thereby increasing the urethral pressure that can help decrease urine leakage [172, 173]. As a result, this exercise can either prevent or treat SUI during pregnancy.

CONCEPTS AND DEFINITIONS OF PELVIC FLOOR MUSCLE EXERCISE

Pelvic floor muscle exercises, also known as Kegel exercises, are the most popular method of treatment for SUI. In the late 1940s, an American gynecologist named Arnold Kegel first introduced this method for treatment of postpartum UI and improving the function and tone of the pelvic floor muscles following childbirth. PFME are successful because postpartum women who have performed these exercises have reported cure rates as high as 84% and improvement rates as high as 100% [174].

At present, PFME is generally accepted as the first-line of treatment for SUI [167] because PFME is a safe means of treatment with no complications. Furthermore, the exercises are inexpensive, require no instruments and can be done anywhere and anytime [168, 169].

The goals of PFME in the treatment of SUI are to strengthen the endurance of the pelvic floor muscles and thereby enhance the urethral closure pressure [175] while elevating the urethrovesicular junction and increasing the tone of the pelvic floor muscles [176].

In addition, the outcomes of PFME not only cure but also improve conditions, prevent complications and offer comfort [177].

Pelvic floor muscle exercises may include active and isometric exercise or static exercise in which the muscle maintains a constant length and contraction against a fixed or immovable object [178].

These exercises should be voluntary maximum contractions resulting in contributions to the strength and endurance of the pelvic floor muscles [179].

Definition of Pelvic Floor Muscle Exercise

The International Continence Society [ICS, 1992] refers to PFME as repetitive selective voluntary contraction and relaxation of specific pelvic floor muscles [180]. The Agency of Health Care Policy and Research [AHCPR, 1996] defines PFME as that performed to strengthen the voluntary muscles between and around the vagina and anus, thereby contributing to the closing force of the urethra and the support of the pelvic organs [181].

According to Johnson [182], PFME refers to alternatively contracting and relaxing the pubococcygeus muscle and is designed to help strengthen the pelvic floor muscles. The National Institute of Health [183] refers to PFME as increasing the strength of the voluntary periurethral and pelvic floor, the contraction of which exerts a closing force on the urethra. Holroy-Ledue and Straus [184] defines PFME as a program of repeated voluntary pelvic floor muscle contractions. In summary, PFME refers to a program of repeated voluntary contractions and relaxation of specific pelvic floor muscles designed to help strengthen and improve the supportive and sphincteric function of the pelvic floor muscle and possibly contributing to the closing force of the urethra and the support of the bladder neck and urethra [185].

Muscles Used in the Pelvic Floor Muscle Exercise

The pelvic organs are supported and suspended by pelvic floor muscles and ligamentous tissues as well as the attachments between muscles, ligaments and the bony pelvis. Voluntary pelvic floor muscle contractions cause a squeeze and inward lift of the pelvic floor muscle with resultant urethral closure, stabilization and resistance to downward movement [186].

The pelvic floor muscles and ligaments play an essential role in the maintenance of UI and can be described as follows:

1. Pelvic Floor Muscles

Pelvic floor muscles are striated muscles comprising the levator ani and coccygeus muscles. The levator ani is a complex muscle that includes the pubococcygeus, puborectalis, and illiococcygeus muscles, through which the urethra, vagina and rectum pass. Different muscles have different fiber directions and each muscle is capable of contracting in isolation [186]. When these muscles are strong, they contract to keep the meatuses closed and maintain urethral closure pressure in what is known as sphincteric function. This is a broad flat muscle forming the anterior part of the pelvic floor and attaching to the bony pelvis, where it acts as a sling to help hold the pelvic organs (urethra, vagina and rectum) in place in its supportive function. Coccygeus is a triangular sheet of muscle and tendinous fibers situated behind the levator ani [186].

The muscle fibers of the pelvic floor muscles contain type I (slow-twitch) fibers and type II (fast-twitch) fibers [66, 187]. The slow-twitch muscle fibers have smaller diameters of muscle fiber than the fast-twitch muscle fibers to assist in improving muscle endurance by generating a slower, more sustained, but less forceful contraction.

In contrast, fast-twitch muscle fibers are capable of very short, but forceful contractions capable of responding to sudden intra-abdominal pressure by contributing to urethral closure pressure [152, 187]. The pelvic floor muscles are composed of approximately 70% slow-twitch and 30% fast-twitch muscle fibers [188].

2. Ligaments

Ligaments are the thickened parts of the endopelvic fascia of the pelvic floor muscle. The ligaments are attached between the bony pelvis and the pelvic organs to support the suspension of the pelvic organs and maintain continence.

For example, the pubrourethral ligament is attached to the mid-urethra; the urethropelvic ligament is attached to the bladder neck and proximal-urethra; and the vescicopelvic ligament is attached to the bladder to help support the bladder neck and keep the urethra in place during intra-abdominal pressure, which can be prevent UI [2].

In summary, the pelvic floor muscles play a major role in supporting the pelvic organs and maintaining urinary continence by two main supportive and sphincteric functions.

In addition, the ligaments are attached to the urethra and bladder neck to support and prevent displacement of the urethra and bladder neck during intra-abdominal pressure occurring with coughing, sneezing, laughing and jumping in order to help prevent UI.

Identification of Correct Pelvic Floor Muscle Contraction

A correct pelvic floor muscle contraction is defined as inward movement with squeezing around the pelvic openings [189, 190]. One barrier to PFME might be deficient knowledge about how to correctly perform pelvic floor muscle contractions [191].

Wilson and Herbison [192] found deficient knowledge about how to correctly perform contractions as the key reason for not practicing PFME in women. Bump et al. [175] found more than 30% of women to be unable to contract pelvic floor muscle correctly at the first consultation.

Similarly, another study by Henderson et al. [193] found 15.4% of women who initially incorrectly contracted the pelvic floor muscle; however, 78% of these women learned after brief instruction.

Most women report knowing about PFME whereby approximately two thirds (65.7%) of women reported feeling very or quite confident about their ability to perform PFME correctly [191]. Consistent with the aforementioned finding, there is some evidence that few women are actually taught how to perform PFME [191, 194].

Henderson et al. [193] reported pelvic floor muscle contractions to be performed correctly on the first attempt in 83.4% of women with SUI, concluding that most women with no or mild pelvic floor disorders can correctly contract pelvic floor muscle after a simple verbal cue; hence, the researchers suggested that PFME can be initiated without clinical confirmation on correct pelvic floor muscle technique.

Before pregnant women with SUI begin PFME, they must be certain they are exercising the correct muscles. Pregnant women, therefore, should receive instructions about identifying the pelvic floor muscles [177] and correctly contracting and relaxing the pelvic floor muscles as follows:

1. Periurethral or Perivaginal Muscle Contraction

Periurethral or perivaginal muscle contraction is an anterior PFME in which pregnant women can imagine that they are trying to stop urine flow or contracting as often experienced during coitus when the vagina clasps the penis [195]. To identify pelvic floor muscle contraction, the pregnant women can try one of the following methods:

1.1. Stop Test

Stop test, or the ability to stop urination promptly and on command, has been shown to be associated with the function of the pelvic floor musculature [196]. During urination, women were asked to sit on the toilet with legs spread wide apart. Begin urinating and, at midstream, try to stop the urine stream by contracting the pelvic floor muscles to clamp down and close the urethra. Hold this contraction to cut off the urine flow for approximately 1-2 seconds, and then relax the muscle to complete urination.

Pregnant women who perform correct pelvic floor muscle contractions will be able to stop the urine flow for a brief moment [182, 197, 198]. Do not perform this stop test on a regular basis or more than once per month as it may be a cause of urinary tract infection. Only use this test as an assessment of the muscle.

1.2. Vaginal Palpation

Vaginal palpation: while reclining on the back in bed with the knees bent up, insert one or two clean fingers into the vagina. Then contract the pelvic floor muscles or the perivaginal muscle. When the muscle is contracted effectively, the muscle will squeeze or clamp down around the fingers and begin to pull them upward [41].

Chiarelli et al. [191] concluded that demonstration of pelvic floor muscle contraction is best done in the context of a vaginal examination. The women should have vaginal examination to assess correct contracts of the pelvic floor muscle [170].

Therefore, nurses in primary care settings who see postnatal women routinely for several reasons such as cervical smears or family planning could use these opportunities to ask about incontinence problems [170].

1.3. Observation

Observation: Pregnant women who continue to have difficulty can recline on the back in bed with knees bent up and feet on the bed. Those who are comfortable using a mirror can directly watch the movement of the vagina for evidence of correct contraction. When the pelvic floor muscles are contracted correctly, the vagina moves slightly toward the inside and the clitoris descends toward the vagina as the rectum pulls inward and upward [152, 195].

2. Anal Sphincter or Perianal Muscle Contraction

Anal sphincter or perianal muscle contraction is a posterior PFME in which pregnant women can imagine they are trying to hold back unwanted passage of intestinal gas [182].

This PFME alternatively contracts and relaxes both the anterior and posterior pelvic floor muscles. Pregnant women who can identify the pelvic floor muscles and perform pelvic floor muscle contractions correctly must remember this muscle and contraction for use in performing PFME.

Therefore, health professionals need to be actively involved in educating and demonstrating to women about how to perform PFME [191]. Moreover, women with SUI are advised to seek medical help before beginning a program of PFME in order to ensure they are first properly educated on contraction techniques [193].

Pregnant women can perform PFME in several positions such as lying, sitting, kneeling and standing positions with legs apart, depending on convenience and preference, to emphasize specific strengthening of the pelvic floor muscles and relaxation of other muscles in the body [41]. Pregnant women are instructed to contract or squeeze the pelvic floor muscles prior to sudden intra-abdominal pressure (known as "knack") occurring with coughing, sneezing and jumping. The knack may help reduce pressure on the pelvic floor muscles as it increases the urethral pressure [199, 200].

Patterns of Pelvic Floor Muscle Exercise

Although PFME is recommended as the most effective conservative treatment for women with SUI, there are only limited indications as to which type of PFME is the most effective [201, 202]. This type of exercise varies in terms of the duration or the length of time of each contraction, the positions in which the exercises are performed, the number of contractions performed per session, the number of sessions performed per day, the duration of exercise and the type of instruction provided [184, 202, 203].

Morkved et al. [41], for example, studied the effects of PFME aimed at preventing UI in nulliparous women with gestational ages of more than 20 weeks. The nulliparous women trained with a physiotherapist for weekly 60-minute sessions over a period of 12 weeks between gestational ages of 20 and 36 weeks. The physiotherapist encouraged the women to perform both slow and fast contractions in which slow contractions involved performing a pelvic floor muscle contraction and holding the contraction for 6-8 seconds followed by a relaxation period of 6 seconds. At the end of each contraction, the women were asked to add three to four fast contractions. The women were encouraged to perform 8 to 12 sets of pelvic floor muscle contractions twice per day at home for a total of 16 to 24 sets per day.

Reilly et al. [159] studied the effects of antenatal PFME in primigravidae women with bladder neck mobility at gestational ages of more than 20 weeks to prevent postpartum SUI. The women were encouraged to perform PFME comprising three sets of eight contractions in which each contraction was held for six seconds followed by two minutes of relaxation of the muscle between sets. These exercises were repeated twice per day. At gestational ages of 34 weeks until delivery, the number of contractions per session was increased to 12. In addition, the women performed supervised PFME with a physiotherapist once a month at hospital from gestational ages of 20 weeks until delivery.

Sampsell et al. [161] studied the effects of PFME on SUI and pelvic floor muscle strength during pregnancy and the postpartum period in 72 primigravidae women with gestational ages of 20 weeks.

The daily recommended number of contractions was 30 at maximum or near maximum intensity for strength building.

Glazener et al. [157] suggested that women perform PFME for ten contractions per set in eight to ten sessions per day of fast and slow contractions for a total of 80-100 contractions per day. This finding suggests that postpartum PFME can reduce the incidence of persistent postpartum UI for up to 12 months postpartum.

Pearson and Kelber [197] suggested that patients perform PFME with both slow and fast contractions as follows: fast contractions are held for 1 second and relaxed for 1 second, then repeated for at total of approximately 10 contractions. Slow contractions involve tightening the pelvic floor muscles and holding contractions for approximately 10 seconds, then relaxing for another 10 seconds and repeating for about 10 sets for a total of 60 contractions per day.

Johnson [182] recommended PFME comprising both quick and slow contractions in which quick or fast contractions involved alternately contracting and relaxing the pelvic floor muscles rapidly whereas slow contractions were performed by tightening the muscles and holding the contraction for three to ten seconds.

The patients were recommended to perform 10 contractions per set in four daily sessions for a total of 40 contractions per day.

AHCPR recommended that women sustain a contraction for at least 10 seconds followed by an equal period of relaxation. These exercises should be performed approximately 30-80 times a day for at least 8 weeks and may need to be continued indefinitely. Elderly people may require a longer period of time to train and condition the muscles to contract with increases in intra-abdominal pressure; the pelvic muscles should be contracted before and during situations involving potential leakage [181].

In conclusion, PFME varies in terms of the duration or length of time of each contraction, the number of contractions performed per set, the number of sessions performed per day, the duration of exercise and the type of instructions provided. Pelvic floor muscle exercise, however, can generally be categorized into two major types, namely, slow and fast contractions, because both slow and fast contractions are appropriate for both slow and fast-twitch muscle fibers [152, 182]. Slow contractions are performed by tightening the pelvic floor muscles and holding the contraction for a certain number of seconds, then relaxing for the same number of seconds. This type of exercise is appropriate for type I or slow-twitch muscle fibers. A fast contraction is a short contraction, rapid relaxation of the pelvic floor muscles patients can perform for approximately 1-2 seconds for each contraction-release of the muscle. The contractions are performed several times per set and are appropriate for type II or fast-twitch muscle fiber. Patients are encouraged to perform this exercise continually for at least 4 weeks, to result in alleviation of SUI symptoms and contribute to the continence mechanism.

Effects of Pelvic Floor Muscle Exercise to Prevent and Treat Stress Urinary Incontinence during Pregnancy

Patient's who perform PFME correctly and continually can help increase the strength and endurance of the pelvic floor muscles. As a result, muscle fiber hypertrophy may occur after specific strengthening exercises for at least 3 to 4 weeks [204, 205]. Hence, pelvic floor muscle strength can improve the supportive function of the bladder neck and urethra as well as the sphincteric function of the external urethral sphincter [152] which can improve or cure SUI symptoms [181].

The various effects of PFME for the treatment or prevention of SUI among pregnant women are listed below.

Sampsell et al. [161] studied the effects of PFME on SUI and pelvic floor muscle strength during pregnancy and the postpartum period in 72 primigravidae women with gestational ages of 20 weeks. This study suggested that PFME can reduce the incidence of SUI at a gestational age of 35 weeks as well as six weeks and six months postpartum by significantly increasing pelvic floor muscle strength. The results of this study found the women who performed PFME to exhibit significantly diminished SUI symptoms at a gestational age of 35 weeks ($F[1,43] = 4.36$, $p = .043$) as well as at 6 weeks ($F[1,43] = 4.94$, $p = .032$) and 6 months postpartum ($F[1,43] = 4.29$, $p = .044$) as compared with the women who did not perform PFME.

Reilly et al. [159] studied the effects of antenatal PFME for the prevention of postpartum SUI in primigravidae women with bladder neck mobility and gestational ages of more than 20 weeks, finding antenatal PFME to be capable of preventing postpartum SUI in primigravidae women with bladder neck mobility. According to the findings, the pregnant women who performed PFME for at least 28 days reported only 19.2% postpartum SUI at 3 months after delivery compared with 32.7% in the control group (RR 0.59, 95% CI 0.37-0.92).

Morkved et al. [41] studied the effects of PFME on the prevention of UI in nulliparous women with gestational ages of more than 20 weeks, finding PFME during pregnancy to be effective at strengthening the pelvic floor muscles and preventing UI during pregnancy and after delivery. The results of this study showed that pregnant women in the experimental group who performed PFME reported 32% UI at a gestational age of 36 weeks as compared to 48% in the control group (p=.007). The number of urinary leakage episodes at the gestational age of 36 weeks was also significantly lower in the experimental group (p=.014). Furthermore, pelvic floor muscle strength was significantly higher in the women in the experimental group who performed PFME at a gestational age of 36 weeks and at 3 months after delivery than in the control group (p=.008 and p=.048, respectively).

Dinc et al. [206] studied the effectiveness of PFME on UI during pregnancy and the postpartum period, conducting a study in 80 pregnant women divided into two groups. The intervention involved having the researcher instruct about how to perform the PFME.

Both groups were evaluated for pelvic floor muscle strength and urinary complaints in their 36th to 38th week of pregnancy and sixth to eighth postpartum weeks. According to the findings, the study group had a significant decrease in UI episodes during pregnancy and in the postpartum period. Furthermore, pelvic floor muscle strength increased to a larger extent.

Hence, it was concluded that PFME are quite effective in the augmentation of the pelvic floor muscle strength and in the treatment of urinary incontinence.

Kocaöz et al. [207] determined the role of PFME in the prevention of SUI during pregnancy and the postpartum period in 102 pregnant women. Both the exercise and control groups were evaluated in terms of SUI at gestational ages of 14, 20, 28, and 32 weeks and at 12 weeks postpartum. As shown by the pad test at the end of the study, SUI developed in 5.8, 17.3 and 1.9% of the women in the intervention group at the 28th and 32nd gestational week and the 12th postpartum week, respectively. The relevant ratios in the control group were 30, 48 and 18 percent, respectively.

A statistically significant difference was found between the intervention and control groups in terms of SUI development at the 28th and 32nd weeks of gestation and the 12th postpartum week ($p < 0.05$). Therefore, this study concluded that PFME was effective for prevention of SUI development during pregnancy and in the postpartum period.

Sangsawang and Serisathien [208], investigated the effects of a PFME on the severity of SUI in 66 pregnant women who had SUI with gestational ages of 20-30 weeks. The main outcome measure was severity of SUI which comprised frequency and amount of urine leakage and perceived severity of SUI. After the PFME program, the severity of SUI in terms of frequency, amount of urine leakage and scores for perceived SUI severity were significantly reduced compared to the same scores before participation in the program. In addition, the pregnant women in the experimental group had frequency, volume of urine leakage and score for perceived SUI severity after participation that were significantly reduced compared to the pregnant women in the control group.

Hence, the researchers concluded that the 6-week PFME program was able to decrease the severity of symptoms in pregnant women with SUI.

Ko et al. [209] evaluated the effects of antenatal PFME in the prevention and treatment of UI during pregnancy and the postpartum period in 300 nulliparous women with gestational ages of 16 to 24 weeks who were randomly assigned to the PFME and control groups. During late pregnancy and the postpartum period, the pregnant women in the PFME group were found to have significantly lower total UDI-6 and IIQ-7 scores.

Moreover, the self-report rate of UI was also less than in the control group. This study concluded that PFME applied in pregnancy is effective in the treatment and prevention of UI during pregnancy; moreover this effect may persist into the postpartum period.

Stafne et al. [210] assessed the effects of a 12-week performed pelvic floor muscle training (PFMT) program aimed at reducing self-reported UI and fecal incontinence (FI) in late pregnancy in 855 pregnant women. The intervention was a 12-week exercise program, including PFMT conducted between 20 and 36 weeks of gestation. One weekly group session was led by physiotherapists, and home exercises were encouraged at least twice a week. The control group received regular antenatal care only. After the intervention, fewer women in the intervention group reported any weekly UI and FI (11% vs. 19%, P=0.004 and 3% vs. 5%, P=0.18, respectively). Hence, it was indicated that pregnant women who perform PFMT can prevent and treat UI in late pregnancy.

Pelaez et al. [211], investigated the effects of pelvic floor muscle training (PFMT) taught in a general exercise class during pregnancy on the prevention of urinary incontinence (UI) in 169 nulliparous continent pregnant women. The participants were randomized by a central computer system to an exercise group (n = 73) or a control group (n = 96). The intervention consisted of 70-75 sessions (22 weeks, three times per week, 55-60 min/session, including 10 min of PFMT), while the control received routine care only (follow up by midwives including information about PFMT). At the end of the intervention, there was a statistically significant difference in favor of the exercise group. The women in the exercise group reported no frequency and leakage of UI 95.2% compared with 60.7% in the control group (P < 0.001, respectively).

Hence, the researchers concluded that PFMT taught in a general exercise class three times per week for at least 22 weeks without former assessment of ability to perform a correct contraction was effective in primary prevention of UI in primiparous pregnant women.

Mason et al. [212], conducted a randomized controlled trial to determine the efficacy of antenatal PFME in the primary prevention of postpartum stress incontinence in primiparous women. Pregnant women were randomized to an intervention (n = 141) or control group (n = 145). The intervention comprised four sessions of PFME training during pregnancy and 8-12 maximal contractions repeated twice daily at home. A modified Bristol Female Lower Urinary Tract Symptom questionnaire, the Leicester Impact Scale, and Three

Day Diary were administered at 20 and 36 weeks of pregnancy and three months postpartum.

According to the findings, the intervention group was more likely to exercise pelvic floor muscles compared to the control group at 36 weeks ($p = 0.019$) and three months (0.022), reporting fewer episodes of incontinence and a lower score on the Leicester Impact Scale. However, these differences were not statistically significant.

In summary, antenatal PFME is not only effective for the prevention and treatment of SUI during late pregnancy and the postpartum period, but can also relieve SUI symptoms. According to the review of literature of the AHCPR about the effects of PFME on SUI, most studies were found to report more than 50% reduction in urinary leakage episodes and 25% reported a 100-percent effective cure [181]. Furthermore, the Cochrane review [171] concluded that pregnant women who exercise with intensive antenatal PFME are 56% less likely to report UI in late pregnancy and 30% less likely during the first six postpartum months than women who do not practice PFME.

PART III: FACTORS RELATED TO INCREASED COMPLIANCE IN PERFORMING PELVIC FLOOR MUSCLE EXERCISES DURING PREGNANCY

PFME is a specific exercise that differs from exercise for other muscles in the body. Thus, PFME requires a strong commitment from both patients and health care professionals. This form of exercise requires dedication, endurance and effort on the part of women to continuously follow PFME protocol in order to result in effective treatment of SUI [152]. Therefore, the adherence to a PFME regimen is an essential factor for the effectiveness of PFME [213].

Unfortunately, several long-term follow-up studies have demonstrated that many women decrease their adherence to PFM exercise over time [213-216]. Barriers, or factors that interfere with PFM exercise adherence, may include poor exercise instruction from health care providers; ambivalence regarding the effectiveness of PFME to prevent and treat SUI; deficient of knowledge about how to perform PFME correctly; forgetting to exercise; no time to exercise; no interest in exercise; no self-motivation to exercise; and interference by daily activities or other illnesses [217-221].

Borello-France et al. [222] found that trouble remembering to exercise was the most frequently reported exercise barrier. Other barriers to performing

PFME reported by women include illness of self or family, vacation/travel, fatigue, work, personal conflicts and boredom with exercise.

Moreover, it has been suggested that the predictors of exercise adherence change over time. Among the many variables examined during supervised intervention, lower baseline UI frequency (<14 UI episodes per week) and higher levels of self-reported mental health (higher SF-36 mental scores) were found to predict exercise adherence.

At three months, lower baseline Brink scores (weaker PFMs) were the only statistically significant predictor of PFM exercise adherence. At 12 months post-randomization, the barrier "having trouble remembering to exercise" was found to be the only statistically significant predictor of PFM exercise adherence.

Conversely, reasonable expectations and flexible recommendations for exercise, affirmation of correct exercise technique and symptom improvement, a desire to avoid surgical treatment and regular follow-up with a health care professional have been identified as factors that promote PFM exercise adherence [218, 220]. The factors influencing the success of PFME can be discussed in greater detail as follows:

1. Age

Older age in women leads to loss of nerve function and decreases in the total number of striated muscle fibers of the urethral sphincter at a rate of 2% a year [85, 86] as well as loss of urethral closure pressure [84]. These findings indicate that the strength of pelvic floor muscle tissue reduces with age. Hence, it may be concluded that older women have less pelvic floor muscle strength than younger women. Therefore, the outcome of PFME in treating and preventing SUI may also be associated with age.

It may be that younger women with stronger muscles experience a stronger sense of muscle and leakage control, and attribute this control to exercise which further leads to sustained adherence.

Conversely, older women with weaker muscles may have less proprioceptive feedback from PFM contractions or lower sense of efficacy, thereby giving these women less reason to sustain their efforts when they are no longer seeing the interventionist [222].

These findings suggest that women with weak muscles should spend more time in initial supervised therapy. Alternatively, the women might be followed periodically to assess PFM control, modify maintenance of the exercise program and support adherence until it is more self-sustained [222].

In addition, Bishop et al. [223] examined the factors affecting pelvic floor muscle response to PFME in 85 women aged 35 to 78 years. The women were encouraged to perform a PFME program beginning with 15 repetitions of holding pelvic floor muscle contractions for 12 seconds each. Ten repetitions were added every 3 weeks for a total of 12 weeks and 45 repetitions by the end of the program.

The findings from the aforementioned program suggest that some older women may drop out from the PFME program before optimal training effects to strengthen the muscle have occurred.

2. Parity and Mode of Delivery

The number of previous deliveries and pregnancies was significantly higher in the incontinent pregnant women than continent pregnant women [27]. Multiparous women are associated with greater risk for SUI than primiparae [46, 91]. In addition, vaginal delivery is well-known to be associated with pelvic floor dysfunction and reduced urethral closure pressure. Furthermore, bladder neck mobility increases significantly after all vaginal births [93], which can develop risks for SUI [97]. Leijonhufvud et al. [99] found the significantly increased risk of SUI later in life among women who had only delivered by vaginal birth compared to those delivering only by cesarean delivery. Therefore, cesarean section could have a protective role in postpartum SUI in comparison to vaginal delivery [105, 106]. These findings may indicate the factors of women with multiparity and vaginal delivery to be associated with increased risk for the development of SUI. Hence, women with potential risk factors for developing SUI are more likely to perform PFME to prevent or treat SUI than women with minimal or no risks.

These findings are supported by Bo et al. [224] who found women regularly performing PFME at six months' postpartum to be women who had more children (2 children adjusted OR = 1.17, $\geq$ 3 children adjusted OR = 1.45). Conversely, those women who delivered by cesarean section were less likely to perform PFME (adjusted OR = 0.56, 95% CI 0.51-0.61).

3. Severity of Stress Urinary Incontinence Symptoms

Women with mild to moderate SUI symptoms may achieve more improvement in incontinence with conservative treatment by PFME compared to those reporting more severe symptoms [183, 225-227]. However, Alewijnse et al. [216] found women with severe symptoms (more frequent wet episodes per week) to be more likely to retain higher adherence to PFME than women with mild to moderate symptoms (less frequent wet episodes per week). This result is consistent with the study of Chen and Tzeng [228] who found greater severity of UI (based on both UI frequency and amount of urine loss) to predict PFM exercise adherence in women with UI who underwent at least 6 weeks of exercise. In another study with similar findings, Mason et al. [229] found women with current UI issues to be more motivated to perform PFME.

It is possible that the amount of urine leakage is a strong predictor of intention to adhere to PFME. Moreover, women who have more frequency of urine leakage are associated with more long-term PFME adherence at 1 year after receiving PFME therapy [216, 230].

For short-term PFME effectiveness, Hung et al. [231] found the effectiveness of a 4-month PFM strengthening program to be influenced by the severity of SUI symptoms instead of exercise adherence.

In addition, the findings of the aforementioned study also indicate that no direct evidence has demonstrated exercise adherence as a significant predictor of PFME effectiveness for women with symptomatic UI.

The aforementioned finding may due to the fact that women with mild symptoms may not perceive their incontinence as a serious problem whereas patients with severe symptoms recognize the incontinence as an ongoing problem and view adherence to exercise as positive training aimed at a cure [232]. Moreover, it is possible that severity of SUI symptoms may influence adherence to PFM exercise differently in women with SUI versus urgency-predominant UI because women with urge or urgency-predominant symptoms typically experience greater volume of urine loss with each leakage episode compared to women with SUI [222].

In contrast, Borello-France et al. [222] reported a higher proportion of women with less frequent UI (<14 UI episodes per week) compared with more frequent UI (>14 UI episodes per week) who were adherent to exercise recommendations (72% versus 59%, P=.02). In the logistic regression model, UI frequency was significantly associated with adherence.

Interestingly, Theofrastous et al. [233] found woman's response to PFME does not depend on the severity of clinical SUI symptoms.

4. Knowledge about Stress Urinary Incontinence and Pelvic Floor Muscle Exercise

Another reason for women not engaging in PFME may be deficient knowledge about PFME [234]. Despite the benefits of PFME in preventing and treating UI in pregnant women, Fine et al. [213] found only 64% of the women in the study to report what they had learned about PFME during pregnancy or the postpartum period.

In addition, Jette et al. [235] reported another reason for non-adherence provided by the women, finding adherence to exercise to be decreased when health professionals are not concerned about explaining the benefits and the rationale of PFME.

Women's belief that PFME is unnecessary in solving their SUI symptoms is the most frequently (69%) reported reason women provide for not performing PFME [213].

Although a high percentage (77.9%) of all pregnant women know about PFME during pregnancy, only three-quarters of pregnant women report access to information about PFME in the current pregnancy [16]. Whitford et al. [16] found a high percentage of younger women, first-time mothers and mothers from more underprivileged groups to be less likely to report having information about PFME. In addition, they also found midwives to be the health professionals most likely to provide information about PFME and books to be the most frequently mentioned source of information.

In a qualitative survey with semi-structured interviews of 42 women conducted by Mason et al. [236], women who had knowledge about UI and received instructions to do PFME were found to be motivated to perform PFME. Mason et al. [203] found 55% of women to have received some form of instruction in pelvic floor exercises by 34 weeks of pregnancy and 86% of women to have received instruction following birth. The type of information provided varied, ranging from a brief reminder to exercising in a class with an instructor. The information was provided by a wide range of health professionals, and no single profession appeared to undertake responsibility for the service. As a result, the views of the service varied. A few women reported that they had received good quality instruction, while others were critical, and a small number reported that they had received no instruction at all. These findings may indicate that counseling and information about possible pelvic floor muscle trauma during pregnancy and delivery occurs significantly less frequently than health education on general topics during pregnancy [237].

5. Knowledge about How to Correctly Perform Pelvic Floor Muscle Exercise

One barrier to PFME adherence is deficient knowledge about how to correctly perform PFME. Wilson and Herbison [192] found deficient knowledge to be a key reason for not performing PFME.

In addition, Chiarelli and Cockburn [194] also found women with inadequate awareness about the required frequency and duration of PFME, rare lessons on how to perform PFME and frequent uncertainty about whether or not PFME is performed correctly. Bo et al. [234] stated that deficient understanding about how to contract the muscles correctly may be another reason among women who fail to complete PFME. In other words, women might confuse PFME with other muscle training such as exercise for the gluteal, hip adductor and abdominal muscles [238].

Chiarelli et al. [191] found that, although most women report knowing about PFME, only 15.7% perform PFME adequately before their most recent pregnancy and slightly over half had performed PFME adequately during pregnancy. In terms of correct PFME performance, approximately two thirds (65.7%) of the women reported feeling very or quite confident about their ability to perform PFME correctly.

It is likely that some of these women did not perform pelvic floor muscle correctly at all [191], possibly indicating that few women are actually taught how to correctly perform PFME, particularly in the context of a per vaginum (PV) examination [194]. Before pregnant women begin PFME, therefore, they must be certain that they are exercising the right muscles [191, 203].

Hilde et al. [38] found 6% of women to report uncertainty about whether they contracted correctly and 8 % to report inability to voluntarily stop the urine stream when voiding to evaluate correct pelvic floor muscle contraction.

It is possible that misunderstanding about how to perform correct pelvic muscle contraction led to reduced effectiveness of PFME in treating UI symptoms. Therefore, all women should receive instruction about this knowledge and evaluated the ability to correctly contract their pelvic floor muscles before starting a PFME program.

6. Insufficient Time

PFME requires a strong commitment from the women in exerting effort to performing PFME in combination with the protocol guidelines in order to result in effective treatment of SUI [152].

Forgetting and being too busy were other common reasons women provided for not performing PFME [213].

Interestingly, Holley et al. [239] suggested deficient time and discipline in performing exercise to also have been reported as reasons for poor long-term PFM adherence in women with SUI.

However, many women may be expected to claim that they are too busy with daily life activities and deem themselves incapable of integrating exercise into their busy lives. Therefore, health professionals who provide the information about PFME to women can state that PFME takes very little time per day and can be performed during any kind of activity without being noticed by other people [230]. Furthermore, women who have no time for regular visits to a physiotherapist could be instructed in PFME by their GPs during consultations.

7. Cooperation

PFME is a specific strength exercise for the pelvic floor muscle and relaxation of other muscles in the body. During this exercise, no other muscles in the body such as the abdominal, back or leg muscles are to be contracted and patients are to breathe normally while exercising [182].

Thus, cooperation, firm commitment and endurance are required from women in order to successfully achieve these exercises. Moreover, health care professionals must recognize and help promote the women's perception of their self-efficacy and the benefits of PFME for the treatment of incontinence.

In this way, incontinent women may gain motivation for adherence to PFME. Unfortunately, MaLennan et al. [237] found nearly-half of pregnant women (46%) received no information about PFME during pregnancy. In addition, pregnant women received less counseling about issues related to pelvic floor dysfunction than instruction about general health care during pregnancy such as high blood pressure, weight gain, or early labor [237].

8. Method of Instruction

Although PFME doesn't require instruments and can be done anywhere and anytime [169], several studies have recommended that exercise in different methods of instruction results in different effects on the treatment of incontinence as well as adherence to PFME. For example, Bo et al. [204]

indicated greater improvement in women who exercised with an instructor once per week for 6 months as compared to women who exercised on their own at home. Similar findings were revealed in the study of Wilson et al. [240] who suggested that women who perform PFME under the supervision of a physiotherapist at the hospital achieved significantly better outcomes as compared to those exercising at home alone. According to the findings of a systematic review by Berghmans et al. [201], women who performed PFME and were trained by a physiotherapist at the hospital were more effective and exhibited greater adherence than those who performed PFME at home alone. In addition, the Cochrane review concluded that an intensive PFME training program conducted by physiotherapists over a period of 8 to 12 weeks showed increasing effectiveness of SUI prevention during pregnancy [241].

Group training for PFME by health care providers at hospital is cost-effective and may offer more motivation for both the therapist and the women. In addition, the postpartum training classes may provide an important meeting place for general health promotion for mother and child [42, 242].

Verbal instruction or education can help improve the effectiveness of PFME for the treatment of incontinence. Furthermore, women who were taught by a teacher or instructor about the anatomy, function and structure of pelvic floor muscles as well as the causes of pelvic floor muscle dysfunction, PFME and identity of pelvic floor muscles and contraction tend to achieve higher efficacy and adherence to PFME than women who perform the exercises alone at home [157, 182, 204, 243].

Teaching, education or giving instruction to pregnant women about SUI and PFME is considered health education. Health education is an interaction process between nurses and patients that differs from general education because it does not only aim to provide knowledge about the particular subject, but also to change the learners' attitudes and behaviors. There are several methods for delivery of education to patients. Therefore, instructors have to choose a teaching method that is suitable for their target learners and the contents they intend to deliver. Generally speaking, teaching methods can be categorized into two major groups as follows:

1. Individual teaching or education involves one-on-one coaching between instructor and learner in which the instructor will accurately understand the learner's problems and requirements.

Both the instructor and learner have opportunities to ask questions or conduct activities in order to achieve the goal of the lesson. This method is suitable for teaching learners with varied backgrounds and directly responds to learner's interests, ability and requirements. However, it requires a lot of time, consumes staff work time and is costly.

2. Group teaching or education is teaching provided to a group of more than 2 target learners. An appropriate number of learners for group teaching would range from 5 to 10 and the advantage of group teaching is opportunity to exchange experiences and opinions which may motivate group members to learn and change their health behaviors. Furthermore, group teaching is cost-effective as well as time-effective because the education is delivered to many learners in one class.

Teaching materials are also important for effective education as they are influential to teaching efficacy and learning achievement.

Teaching materials include all materials, equipment and techniques that contain useful information and contents designed to enhance understanding and facilitate learning. Teaching materials are used as media for the effective transfer of knowledge, experience, attitude and skills from an instructor to a learner, thereby leading to learning and changes in health behaviors as determined in the teaching objectives.

There are several types of teaching materials available and the instructor must choose appropriate materials according to each type of education. The various roles of teaching materials in education are listed below:

1 Stimulating and attracting learner's attention, possibly helping to encourage continual participation in the lesson.
2 Improving the effectiveness of learning to help slow learners learn more quickly and easily as they require less time to understand.
3 Assisting with additional instruction by reviewing the lesson for clear understanding.
4 Enhancing knowledge, experience and skills in the activity performance of learners.
5 Decreasing the period of time spent in instruction to allow increased time for other educational activities such as demonstrations, role plays, discussion, etc.

Newman [152] recommended that teaching or verbal instruction are not adequate for teaching incontinent women how to perform PFME, thus indicating that both verbal and non-verbal instruction are essential for teaching women to perform correct PFME.

Non-verbal education may include a booklet or handbook specifically designed for the intervention and re-enforces the verbal instruction in a form the incontinent women easily take back home for unlimited personal review.

In addition, it is more effective to actually perform PFME than to listen to verbal instruction alone [201, 203].

For example, Chiarelli and Cockburn [243] conducted a randomized controlled trial study examining the effects of PFME for the prevention of postpartum urinary incontinence.

The postpartum women were taught and encouraged to perform PFME at home daily and exercised with a physiotherapist at the hospital in addition to receiving a booklet about UI and PFME. The results of this study showed that the women in the experimental group exhibited significantly reduced incidence of UI after childbirth and less severity of UI compared to the women in the control group who received routine care only.

Part IV: Role of Midwives in Promoting Pregnant Women in the Prevention and Treatment of Stress Urinary Incontinence during Pregnancy

Several researchers and a Cochrane systematic review concluded that PFME resulted in improved strength of the pelvic floor muscle during pregnancy and after delivery. Furthermore, the findings indicate that success was dependent on the adherence and correction of muscle contraction. However, this exercise may be inappropriate in real clinical situations. The program of instruction did not meet the recommendations made in the literature. Moreover, it is likely that the success of the randomized controlled trials reported in the literature would not be repeated in the `real world' [203].

In addition, most studies have found that instruction provided by physical therapists might not be suitable for actual implementation in pregnant women because most pregnant women who seek antenatal care do not see physical therapists. In reality, only a very small minority of pregnant women see physical therapists.

Although PFME can be implemented to prevent SUI in continent pregnant women who regularly perform PFME and treat these symptoms in incontinent women, it is impractical for all women to receive supervised PFMT from a physiotherapist or continence advisor in pregnancy [62].

Mason et al. [203] suggested that inadequate instruction about pelvic floor exercises by health professionals may be a problem for many women after delivery. However workload might be a barrier to implementation [62].

Although interventions from various studies finding successful experiences in preventing or treating SUI in pregnant women to not actually be implemented in the care of pregnant women. However, many women thought the information on stress incontinence should be provided during pregnancy because they felt it was important for women to be warned that the condition could occur during pregnancy and the postpartum period [236]. In addition, those women also wanted health professionals to seek out information about symptoms rather than having the women themselves broach the subject [236].

Unfortunately, many instances have shown that not all women receive instruction about SUI and PFME during the antenatal or postnatal periods. It can, therefore, be assumed that a large proportion of women do not receive detailed instruction in pelvic floor exercises [203].

For example, Mason et al. [236] found the majority of women to have not received instruction about SUI either during pregnancy or the postpartum period. However, many women thought information on stress incontinence should be provided during pregnancy because they felt it was important for women to be warned that the condition could occur during pregnancy and the postpartum period [236]. In addition, those women also wanted health professionals to seek out information about symptoms, rather than the women themselves having to broach the subject [236].

Fine et al. [213] found less than one-half of pregnant women to have received instructions from their doctors or midwives. Most instructions were provided verbally, and only 10% of those who received instructions indicated they had had the opportunity to demonstrate a contraction during a pelvic examination. In addition, only approximately one-quarter of the women indicated that they had received instructions before and after childbirth [213].

Mason et al. [203] found few women to have the opportunity to practice alongside a supervisor, even though research suggests that a better outcome is obtained when this is the case. Women report the information provided during antenatal classes to be the best source of information for the following reasons: the information was provided during the last trimester; the instruction was usually detailed and the women were usually given the opportunity to practice the exercises alongside an instructor who could answer any questions, if necessary [203].

In contrast, Whitford et al. [16] found the majority of pregnant women to report being given or obtaining information about pelvic floor exercises during pregnancy and approximately one-third of those women reported receiving information in a parent education class. Books were the most frequently mentioned source of information and midwives were the health professionals most likely to give information about pelvic floor exercises. In addition, the women who had been to classes were significantly more likely to know about the exercises. This information route seems to be effective in communicating the message about pelvic floor exercises [16].

Again, women need to know the effects of PFME on the pelvic floor and the way in which improved pelvic floor muscle function can alleviate SUI symptoms [191]. Therefore, the recommendations suggest that all women be provided information about SUI and how to perform PFME during the antenatal and postnatal periods [236, 244]. Concerning knowledge about PFME, however, the women also need to be informed that PFME are relevant to all phases of life, not only the antenatal period or childbirth years [191].

In fact, the high prevalence of incontinence during pregnancy that increases with gestational age until delivery should not be ignored by all health professionals. Furthermore, detailed inquiry should be made into continence during pregnancy [16]. Therefore, health professionals caring for women during pregnancy or the postpartum period need to raise awareness about SUI [236].

It is well known that physiotherapy encompasses exercise and muscle strengthening programs that are particularly relevant to female urinary incontinence interventions. Moreover, most physiotherapists are trained in these exercises [245]. In Australia, it is advantageous that the majority of Australian hospitals have funded physiotherapists, and physiotherapists are well-placed to deliver this program intervention to women in the hospital setting, as well as later during the postpartum period [245].

In some unfortunate hospitals where physiotherapists are not available, midwives and GPs involved in the care of postpartum women could be trained to deliver this intervention in women to prevent and treat UI [245].

The instruction about pelvic floor exercises could be made explicit in the policies and protocols governing practices, not left to the discretion of the individual career [203]. An `optimal' exercise program could be designed and adopted by all health instructors [246], suggesting the incorporation of at least 2 individual exercise instruction sessions in antenatal/postnatal care.

Similar to the study of Bo et al. [234], no single health professional appeared to undertake responsibility for giving systematic information regarding the importance of performing PFME during pregnancy [234]. This means that pregnant women may receive information regarding bladder control from several health care professionals such as primary care physicians, obstetricians, midwives and leaders of antenatal classes. Therefore, to ensure that women receive accurate and consistent information and advice, efforts should be made to educate healthcare professionals about SUI and PFME, particularly among those practitioners who have most contact with women [191]. These health care professionals need to be regularly updated with new information and encouraged to communicate with one another in the ongoing care of women over the lifespan [191].

As previously mentioned above, most research has been found to demonstrate that pregnant women receive information about SUI and PFME from a number for medical personnel such as midwives, doctors, physiotherapists or GPs, thereby showing duty of providing this information to pregnant women is not exclusive to any particular person. However, the duty should belong to all medical personnel providing care for women during pregnancy, which also includes midwives or nurses. Therefore, midwives, who are considered to be medical personnel most closely working with pregnant women, should apply this information to the care of all pregnant women and part of this role should also be adjusted to nursing practice as follows:

1. Midwives Should Adjust Personal Attitudes or Perspectives Concerning Stress Urinary Incontinence during Pregnancy

Midwives need to first admit that SUI frequently encountered during pregnancy is not a normal condition.

Rather, SUI is an abnormal condition. If encountered in any woman during pregnancy with no risks for weakening the pelvic floor muscles, PFME will help minimize risks and be able to prevent SUI during pregnancy.

2. Midwives Should Be Well-Informed about Stress Urinary Incontinence and Pelvic Floor Muscle Exercise

Midwives should possess knowledge about SUI and SUI prevention by various methods, particularly treatment by PFME which is accepted as the best method for preventing and treating SUI during pregnancy in order to enable the provision of accurate information for pregnant women in the future.

3. Midwives Should Adjust Their Duties and Accept That the Provision of This Information to Pregnant Women Is a Part of Their Regular Work

Midwives should adjust the methods employed in providing information about SUI and PFME as suitable for the characteristics of regular daily work, possibly beginning by screening for SUI risk factors for all pregnant women receiving antenatal services in order to assess which pregnant women are at risk for developing SUI during pregnancy. In addition, midwives should provide additional instruction about SUI and PFME as another topic apart from the instructions for self-care during pregnancy for subjects in which every pregnant woman should instruction such as nutrition, adequate rest, exercise and keeping antenatal appointments.

In this way, the guidelines for providing instruction about SUI and PFME would be easily provided without disturbing the regular workloads of midwives because implementation would only involve adding this content to the content midwives already regularly provide for pregnant women.

Sangi-Haghpeykar et al. [244] suggested that the routine and universal counseling concerning risks for SUI and the efficacy of PFME should become an integral part of antenatal or postpartum care before hospital discharge, emphasizing the importance of designing an exercise program that can be incorporated easily into the daily routines of new mothers [246].

The instruction could be provided routinely as part of antenatal care rather than during antenatal or other voluntary classes attended only by a proportion of the women. The responsibility for the task may be best held by the midwives as they provide care for women during pregnancy when the women suggest information should be given. However, it could be useful to adopt a multidisciplinary approach with respect to reminding women to perform pelvic floor exercises.

4. Correct Misunderstandings about Stress Urinary Incontinence in Pregnant Women and Motivate Pregnant Women to Seek Assistance from Healthcare Professionals

Midwives should correct misunderstandings about SUI in pregnant women who understand that SUI is a normal occurrence during pregnancy that will disappear postpartum without seeking treatment, or that SUI is either unavoidable or untreatable.

Therefore, if midwives discover any pregnant women to have symptoms of SUI, the midwives should advise the pregnant women that having SUI is neither embarrassing nor disgusting. Hence, pregnant women should not be embarrassed about receiving consultation from health care professionals or avoid treatment for the symptoms occurring. Pregnant women should choose to consult health care professionals they trust or feel comfortable about sharing this information with. Midwives are ready to provide this information to all pregnant women.

Most women are reluctant to seek help for treatment of SUI [170]. There are two main reasons for women's reluctance to seek help [236]. First, the women feel they do not need help (or do not want to admit they need help). Some women report that the condition causes no problems [236], believing SUI to be a normal consequence of childbirth [247]. Therefore they had no reason to seek help.

Second, the women did not want to discuss the condition with a health care professional [236]. The women regard the condition as something of a taboo and are embarrassed by having it and, in many cases, talking about it. Therefore, some women are reluctant to discuss their condition with some health professionals, but they would welcome the opportunity to discuss their problem with someone [236].

Alewijnse et al. [230] found the majority of women with UI to fail to seek help due to feelings of shame, deficient knowledge about management options or viewpoints that UI is an inevitable condition after delivery with symptoms increasing with age. Thus, it is important that health professionals ask about symptoms of SUI if women have potential risk factors for developing SUI.

The reluctance to seek professional help appears to be exacerbated by the nature of the women's relationships with some health professionals and a minority of women feel that certain health professionals, usually their GPs, are unapproachable [236]. Other women worry about their reaction, assuming that their condition will be perceived as a minor problem and a waste of their GP's time [236].

Unfortunately, studies exploring doctors' responses to consultation for incontinence also show their response to be unsatisfactory, even with older women and other types of incontinence [236]. These findings may suggest that health professionals needed to initiate the conversation. When health professionals make general enquiries after a women's health, it is seen as a polite gesture to approach conversation about stress incontinence [236].

In addition, the GP does not seem to be the choice of the women to discuss such topics as stress incontinence [236].

Sangi-Haghpeykar et al. [244] found most women do not readily disclose information regarding incontinence to their medical provider. Therefore, health professionals such as the midwife should be identified as the main care provider during the antenatal and postnatal periods [236].

For the participants' preference of personal sources for help with UI, the discussion about SUI is a private issue for women who feel most comfortable discussing SUI with nurses or midwives [44] and find midwives to be the health care professionals who most commonly provided women with information about UI (33%) and PFME (55%).

In addition, women generally perceive the information as being helpful in which the information from physiotherapists obtained the highest mean ratings for helpfulness [44]. It would seem that nurses or midwives need to take responsibility for giving women this information as a matter of routine postpartum care.

Participants indicate group classes to be their least preferred form of help. Therefore, it may be best for health care professionals to raise the topic of UI in private consultations with pregnant and postpartum women [44].

Whitford et al. [16] found few women (21.8%) to report having received information about pelvic floor exercises during pregnancy from a midwife, possibly because midwives regard the encouragement to perform pelvic floor exercises as the recommendation of the physiotherapist. Only 8.4% of women report receiving information from a physiotherapist (not including women who gained information from a physiotherapist during a parent education class).

Generally, women have no contact with a physiotherapist during pregnancy (except when they attend parent education classes or have a physical problem necessitating referral). Consequently, women do not receive this information [16].

In addition, women in the postpartum period indicate that they would also prefer to consult with continence nurses or general nurses if they experienced UI. Health care professionals do not consistently provide postpartum women with information on UI and PFME [44].

This means discussing issues in such a way that pregnant women feel comfortable discussing adherence problems with the midwives.

Therefore, it is pleasing that most research demonstrates that pregnant women perceive midwives are health professionals to whom they are most likely to be able to disclose information or seek consultations about SUI.

5. Instruction about Stress Urinary Incontinence in Pregnancy

In cases where pregnant women come to consult and request information about SUI, midwifes should informed the women about SUI concerning issues such as normal structure, function of the lower urinary tract, prevalence of SUI during pregnancy, pathophysiology of SUI during pregnancy, factors increasing the risk of developing SUI among pregnant women, investigation and assessment of SUI and the impact of urinary incontinence on the quality of life of pregnant women. This information is explained in greater detail in Part I. In addition, if any pregnant women are found to have risk factors for developing SUI during pregnancy, these women should be advised to minimize those risks. Furthermore, some cases might be referred to an expert such as a urogynecologist or physiotherapist, if necessary.

Midwives should not assume that pelvic floor exercises are the duty of physiotherapists, or that pelvic floor exercises will be taught in classes [16]. Midwives need to be more proactive in routinely providing instruction about pelvic floor exercises as they are in a position to target the groups of women who may currently may miss information [16].

New evidence exists for the presence of risk groups for development of SUI, and this highlights the need for identification of these risk factors as part of routine antenatal care [62]. Preventative strategies can now be undertaken including taking a history in the antenatal clinic for pre-pregnancy and antenatal incontinence and referring such women for supervised PFME during both the antenatal and postnatal periods [62]. Pregnancy itself and several risk factors are associated with increased risk for the development of SUI during pregnancy [52, 137]. These risk factors include age, obesity, smoking, constipation, pre-pregnancy SUI and gestational diabetes mellitus in which no association has been found between each risk factor [137].

Pregnant women may have only one risk factor or multiple combined risk factors for developing SUI [137]. The awareness of these circumstances gives the midwife an opportunity to be extra attentive in certain cases where the above mentioned risk factors are present [248]. The midwife should identify high risk pregnancy in all women as described above, and women who have potential risk factors for developing SUI should receive an appropriate diagnosis and adequate treatment [248]. In cases where pregnant women who have risk factors for developing SUI during pregnancy, midwives should advise the women to reduce these risks. For example, obesity is another risk factor for the development of SUI during pregnancy.

Many studies have reported that weight loss can reduce the risk of SUI in women [249-251], but pregnant women who are obese or have high BMI should not lose weight.

Therefore, midwives should advise that prenatal care be increased to an appropriate weight meeting recommendations for total weight gain. According to the Institute of Medicine [252] on the recommended weight gain during pregnancy, a normal weight gain is 11.5-16 kg during pregnancy in women with normal BMI of 18.5-24.9 kg/m^2. For women with a BMI of 25-29.9 kg/m^2, weight gain should not exceed 7-11.5 kg during pregnancy.

And in obese women with a BMI of 30 kg/m^2 or more, weight gain should increase by approximately 7 kg during pregnancy [252].

In this respect, the midwife has an independent role that allows her to act as a detective in identifying women with SUI [248].

In some cases, midwives should collaborate with and refer to urogynecologists, physiotherapists or continence advisors who specialize in the field of PFME therapy, which would be of great value in the outcomes of SUI symptom management [62, 230, 248].

Several researchers concluded that PFME resulted in improved strength of the PFM during pregnancy with effective prevention and treatment of antenatal SUI. PFME is a low-cost, simple treatment but must be properly initiated [248]. If the midwife has knowledge about SUI and PFME with the ability to alleviate SUI symptoms for women with SUI, the midwife's role can be of great advantage [248].

Concerning the methods of delivering the information to women, a Cochrane review found women who had received regular supervision and follow-up by healthcare professionals who instructed their women to perform PFME and monitored their progress to be more likely to report improvement and adherence than women performing PFME with little or no supervision [172]. However, although the quality and timing of the information at these classes appeared to be good, they are not accessible or accessed by all women [203].

Although research suggests that a better outcome is obtained when this is the case, few women have the opportunity to practice alongside a supervisor.

Therefore, the instruction is usually detailed and the women are usually given the opportunity to practice the exercises alongside an instructor who can answer any questions, if necessary [203].

While the midwife may very well suggest this treatment by providing instruction, the instruction should probably be performed in a clinical setting because it appears that only verbal instructions are insufficient [248].

Importantly, the instruction could be given both verbally and visually while providing women with the opportunity to ask any questions about their symptoms [203].

For visual instruction, the additional distribution of a handbook should be continued as this is an important source of information. The profile of pelvic floor exercises should be raised in other information sources such as magazines, TV and increasingly popular internet websites [16].

6. Providing PFME Instruction

Once pregnant women are armed with knowledge about SUI, the next step midwives should take is to provide instruction about SUI with particular emphasis on PFME, which is the best method for preventing and treating SUI during pregnancy.

Providing instruction at this stage should not focus on teaching through only verbal communication. Rather, both verbal and non-verbal communication should be used together, for example, by teaching aimed at gaining about PFME and correct methods for performing PFME. At this stage, verbal communication might be used.

As for the step of informing patients about whether or not they are able to perform PFME correctly, the pregnant women might need to attend an antenatal class. Lastly, once the pregnant women are confident they are able to perform PFME correctly and will begin doing so in line with PFME protocol once they return home, the pregnant women should receive booklets or handbooks (non-verbal communication). The booklets or handbooks should be composed of the same content the pregnant women have already learned about during the instruction by nurses in order to allow the pregnant women to review the content at home. For knowledge about PFME, pregnant women need to be informed that PFME are relevant to all phases of life, not just the antenatal period or childbirth years. The women also need to know the effects of PFME on the pelvic floor and the way in which improved pelvic floor muscle function can alleviate SUI symptoms [191].

The instruction about SUI and PFME provided for pregnant women should incorporate the following [229]: an explanation as to why PFME is recommended, emphasis on the need to undertake regular and frequent exercise, checking to ensure that women are exercising the right muscles and cues to action in order to help women remember to exercise on a regular basis [229].

PFME cannot be effective if it is not correctly performed [.[213 Therefore, the women need to be shown how to do PFME correctly and encouraged to perform PFME regularly. Health professionals need to be actively involved in educating and demonstrating to women about how to perform PFME as well as encouraging the women to adhere to recommended PFME regimens [191].

However, Bump et al. [175] and Bo et al. [238] found only approximately one-third of women to perform an ideal pelvic floor muscle contraction after brief written or verbal instruction.

The recommendations suggest that all women should be advised to perform PFME during the antenatal and postnatal periods. The women need to be shown how to do PFME correctly and then encouraged to perform PFME regularly. To ensure correct pelvic floor muscle contraction, the recommendations caution against providing women only written instruction [246]. For example, Bump et al. [175] suggested that verbal or written information alone may be inadequate to ensure that women know how to perform the exercises correctly.

The aforementioned findings indicate that clinical assessment of pelvic floor muscle function, assessment of the ability to contract and PFME need to be implemented in antenatal health care. Furthermore, health professionals need to be regularly provided with new scientific knowledge about pelvic floor muscle and PFME [38]. Mason et al. [203] found few women in their study to have received a follow-up to ensure that they were exercising the correct muscles. Those women reported that they were not sure if they were doing the exercises correctly whilst others specially requested that a health professional check whether or not they were performing the exercises properly. Therefore, the women need to ascertain their ability to perform an effective pelvic muscle contraction before starting on a regimen of exercise [203]. Instructors could be made aware of the difficulty women have isolating the correct muscle group; they could also avoid contracting the abdominal, gluteal or thigh muscles, which could be emphasized in addition to the need to avoid `bearing down'. The instruction could incorporate a check to ensure that each woman can perform an effective pelvic floor contraction.

There are several methods for evaluating the ability to contract pelvic floor muscle correctly as described above.

For the women who received the instruction about pelvic floor exercises during pregnancy, a non-invasive technique may be the most appropriate method of verifying a correct muscle contraction [203]. Because midwives are not specially trained to deal with SUI during pregnancy, this follow-up should preferably be as easy and standardized as possible.

It has been advocated that a simple physical examination may reveal SUI [248]. The stop test, however, may be appropriate for midwives in determining the degree of SUI symptoms and testing the ability to correct PFM contractions. In addition, the midwife may also provide the stop test procedure to evaluate the function of the pelvic floor musculature and estimate the strength of the pelvic floor muscle [196, 253].

Vaginal palpation is another muscle evaluation method used by many experts. If the exercises are being taught during pregnancy, a less invasive check such as self palpation may be more appropriate and acceptable to the women. The `optimal' exercise program provided to pregnant women would appear to include both sustained and maximal contractions with regular sessions of exercise per day or several times per week.

A gradual schedule in which women can build up their muscle strength and endurance according to differing abilities may be the most effective means of exercising the pelvic floor.

However, the demonstration of pelvic floor muscle contraction may best be performed in the context of per vagina examination during follow-up in postpartum period. The postpartum visit is an opportune time for the provider to ask about PFME adherence, inquire about any barriers possibly interfering with PFME and confirm during the pelvic examination that the women can perform a correct pelvic floor muscle contraction [213].

Chiarelli et al. [245] found the majority of women ((%72to report no embarrassment in receiving a per vagina examination during the postpartum period while only %5 of those women reported per vagina examination to be quite or extremely embarrassing. It is impossible that most women appear to be more particularly receptive to per vagina examinations during the postpartum period. Most of the women in the study had attended a six-week postpartum check-up which provided an ideal opportunity for a per vagina assessment. Moreover, few women were embarrassed about PFM function testing during per vagina examinations [245]. Thus, health professionals should be informed and reassured that women are likely to be receptive to pelvic floor muscle function testing during the postpartum period, and that the postpartum period is an ideal opportunity for done this assessment [245].

CONCLUSION

The number of pregnant women with SUI is vary, its prevalence ranges from 18.6% to 75% and increases with gestational age.

Both hormonal changes during pregnancy and the commonly encountered physiological changes during pregnancy such as the increasing pressure of the expanding uterus and the fetal weight on the pelvic floor muscle throughout pregnancy may lead to reduced strength of the pelvic floor muscle which has further effect to the supportive function of the bladder neck and the urethra as well as the sphincteric function of the external urethral sphincter. When the urethral pressure becomes less than bladder pressure and intra-abdominal pressure, this is resulted in urethral sphincter incompetence.

Hence, when intra-abdominal pressure is increased during physical activities such as coughing, sneezing, laughing or moving, the pressure inside the bladder becomes greater than the urethral closure pressure. If the urethral sphincter is not strong enough to close the urethra, the consequence is SUI.

SUI during pregnancy is associated with a lack of pelvic floor muscle strength. Therefore, any factors causing weakening of pelvic floor muscle strength are likely to be causal factors for SUI during pregnancy. Several factors such as age, obesity, smoking, constipation, pre-pregnancy SUI and gestational diabetes mellitus may decrease the strength of pelvic floor muscle in addition to pregnancy itself. Pregnant women do not need to have all of the risk factors in order to develop SUI during pregnancy.

Pregnant women may have only one or combination of multiple risk factors to cause SUI. The multiple risk factors may have additive effects to the lack of pelvic floor muscle strength which is increasing the possibility of developing SUI during pregnancy.

PFME by alternately contracting and relaxing the pelvic floor muscle are the most commonly recommended conservative therapy for women with SUI. PFME is aimed to strengthen the pelvic floor and periurethral muscles to improve the continence mechanism.

As a result, this method can either prevent or treat SUI. Several researchers and a Cochrane systematic review have concluded that PFME was resulted in improved strength of the pelvic floor muscle during pregnancy and after delivery. Furthermore, these findings indicate that the successfulness depend on the adherence and correction of muscle contraction. The adherence to a PFME regimen is essential for the effectiveness of PFME.

Unfortunately, several long-term follow-up studies have demonstrated that many women decrease their adherence to PFME over time.

Barriers, or factors that interfere with PFME adherence, may include poor exercise instruction from health care providers; ambivalence regarding the effectiveness of PFME to prevent and treat SUI; deficient knowledge about how to perform PFME correctly; forgetting to exercise; no time to exercise; no interest in exercise; no self-motivation to exercise; and interference by daily activities or other illnesses. However, the success of the randomized controlled trials reported in the literature would not be repeated in the 'real world'. The program of instruction of PFME in real clinical situations did not meet the recommendations made in the literature.

In addition, most studies have found that instruction provided by physiotherapists might not be suitable for actual implementation in pregnant women because most pregnant women who seek antenatal care do not see physiotherapists. In reality, only a very small minority of pregnant women see physiotherapists.

Unfortunately, in some hospitals where physiotherapists are not available, the midwives and GPs who involved in the care of pregnant women could be trained to deliver this intervention to pregnant women to prevent and treat UI. Therefore, no single health professional appeared to undertake responsibility for giving systematic information regarding the importance of performing PFME during pregnancy.

This means that pregnant women may receive information regarding to PFME from several health care profession such as primary care physicians, obstetricians, midwives and the leaders of antenatal classes.

Therefore, midwives, who are considered to be medical personnel most closely working with pregnant women, should apply this instruction to the care of all pregnant women and part of this role should also be adjusted to nursing practice as follows: 1) midwives should adjust personal attitudes or perspectives concerning SUI during pregnancy; 2) midwives should be well-informed about SUI and PFME; 3) midwives should adjust their duties and accept that the provision of this information to pregnant women is a part of their regular work; 4) correct misunderstandings about SUI in pregnant women and motivate pregnant women to seek assistance from healthcare professionals; 5) instruction about SUI in pregnancy and 6) providing PFME instruction to all pregnant women.

To ensure that pregnant women receive accurate and consistent information, efforts should be made to educate healthcare professionals about SUI and PFME, particularly among those practitioners who have most contact with pregnant women.

These health care professionals need to be regularly updated with new information and encouraged to communicate with others in the ongoing care of women over the lifespan.

REFERENCES

[1] Haylen, B. T., de Ridder, D., Freeman, R. M., et al. (2010). An International Urogynecological Association (IUGA)/International Continence Society (ICS) joint report on the terminology for female pelvic floor dysfunction. *Int. Urogynecol. J.*, 21, 5-26.

[2] Delancey, J. O. (2010). Why do women have stress urinary incontinence? *Neurourol. Urodyn.*, 29(Suppl. 1), S13-17.

[3] Ashton-Miller, J. A., Howard, D. and DeLancey, J. O. (2001). The functional anatomy of the female pelvic floor and stress continence control system. *Scand. J. Urol. Nephrol. Suppl.*, 207, 1-12.

[4] Norton, P. and Brubaker, L. (2006). Urinary incontinence in women. *Lancet*, 367(9504), 57-67.

[5] Mangera, A., Patel, A. K. and Chapple, C. R. (2011). Pathophysiology of urinary incontinence. *Surgery*, 29(6), 249-253.

[6] Andersson, K. E. (2004). Detrusor contraction-focus on muscarinic receptors. *Scand. J. Urol. Nephrol. Suppl.*, 215, 54-57.

[7] DeLancey, J. O. (1994). Structural support of the urethra as it relates to stress urinary incontinence: the hammock hypothesis. *Am. J. Obstet. Gynecol.*, 170, 1713-1720.

[8] Blok, B. F. and Holstege, G. (1999). The central control of micturition and continence: implications for urology. *BJU Int.*, 83(suppl. 2), 1-6.

[9] Schytt, E., Lindmark, G. and Waldenstrom, U. (2004). Symptoms of stress incontinence 1 year after childbirth: prevalence and predictors in a national Swedish sample. *Acta Obstet. Gynecol. Scand.*, 83, 928-936.

[10] Viktrup, L. and Lose, G. (2001). The risk of stress incontinence 5 after first delivery. *Am. J. Obstet. Gynecol.,* 185(1), 82-87.

[11] Thom, D. H. and Rortveit, G. (2010). Prevalence of postpartum urinary incontinence: a systematic review. *Acta Obstet. Gynecol. Scand.*, 89(12), 1511-1522.

[12] Wesnes, S. L., Rortveit, G., Bø, K., and Hunskaar, S. (2007). Urinary incontinence during pregnancy. *Obstet. Gynecol.*, 109(4), 922-928.

[13] Mørkved, S. and Bø, K. (1999). Prevalence of urinary incontinence during pregnancy and postpartum. *Int. Urogynecol. J. Pelvic Floor Dysfunct.*, 10, 394-398.

[14] Mason, L., Glenn, S., Walton, I., and Appletion, C. (1999). The prevalence of stress incontinence during pregnancy and following delivery. *Midwifery*, 15(2), 120-128.

[15] Diez-Itza, I., Ibañez, L., Arrue, M., Paredes, J., Murgiondo, A., and Sarasqueta, C. (2009). Influence of maternal weight on the new onset of stress urinary incontinence in pregnant women. *Int. Urogynecol. J. Pelvic Floor Dysfunct.*, 20(10), 1259-1263.

[16] Whitford, H. M., Alder, B. and Jones, M. (2007). A cross-sectional study of knowledge and practice of pelvic floor exercises during pregnancy and associated symptoms of stress urinary incontinence in North-East Scotland. *Midwifery*, 23(2), 204-217.

[17] Huebner, M., Antolic, A. and Tunn, R. (2010). The impact of pregnancy and vaginal delivery on urinary incontinence. *Int. J. Gynecol. Obstet.*, 110(3), 249-251.

[18] Viktrup, L., Lose, G., Rolff, M., and Barford, K. (1992). The symptom of stress incontinence caused by pregnancy or delivery in primiparas. *Obstet. Gynecol.*, 79, 945-949.

[19] Zhu, L., Li, L., Lang, J. H., and Xu, T. (2012). Prevalence and risk factors for peri- and postpartum urinary incontinence in primiparous women in China: a prospective longitudinal study. *Int. Urogynecol. J.*, 23(5), 563-572.

[20] Liang, C. C., Chang, S. D., Lin, S. J., and Lin, Y. J. (2012). Lower urinary tract symptoms in primiparous women before and during pregnancy. *Arch. Gynecol. Obstet.*, 285(5), 1205-1210.

[21] Sun, M. J., Chen, G. D., Chang, S. Y., Lin, K. C., and Chen, S. Y. (2005). Prevalence of lower urinary tract symptoms during pregnancy in Taiwan. *J. Formos. Med. Assoc.*, 104(3), 185-189.

[22] Chittacharoen, A. (2005, January). Urinary and fecal incontinence before and during pregnancy: prevalence and associated factors. *Paper presented at the 19th annual meeting of the Asian and Oceanic Congress of Obstetrics and Gynecology,* Seoul, Korea, October 1-5, 2005.

[23] Sharma, J. B., Aggarwal, S., Singhal, S., Kumar, S., and Roy, K. K. (2008). Prevalence of urinary incontinence and other urological problems during pregnancy: a questionnaire based study. *Arch. Gynecol. Obstet.*, 279(6), 845-851.

[24] Al-Mehaisen, L. M., Al-Kuran, O., Lataifeh, I. M., et al. (2009). Prevalence and frequency of severity of urinary incontinence symptoms in late pregnancy: a prospective study in the north of Jordan. *Arch. Gynecol. Obstet.*, 279(4), 499-503.

[25] Thomason, A. D., Miller, J. M. and Delancey, J. O. (2007). Urinary incontinence symptoms during and after pregnancy in continent and

incontinent primiparas. *Int. Urogynecol. J. Pelvic Floor Dysfunct.*, 18 (2), 147-151.

[26] Raza-Khan, F., Graziano, S., Kenton, K., Shott, S., and Brubaker, L. (2006). Peripartum urinary incontinence in a racially diverse obstetrical population. *Int. Urogynecol. J. Pelvic Floor Dysfunct.*, 17(5), 525-530.

[27] Martins, G., Soler, Z. A., Cordeiro, J. A., Amaro, J. L., and Moore, K. N. (2010). Prevalence and risk factors for urinary incontinence in healthy pregnant Brazilian women. *Int. Urogynecol. J.*, 21(10), 1271-1277.

[28] Brown, S. J., Donath, S., MacArthur, C., McDonald, E. A., and Krastev, A. H. (2010). Urinary incontinence in nulliparous women before and during pregnancy: prevalence, incidence, and associated risk factors. *Int. Urogynecol. J.*, 21(2), 193-202.

[29] Chiarelli, P. and Campbell, E. (1997). Incontinence during pregnancy. Prevalence and opportunities for continence promotion. *Aust. N. Z. J. Obstet. Gynaecol.*, 37(1), 66-73.

[30] Bø, K., PauckØglund, G., Sletner, L., Mørkrid, K., and Jenum, A. (2012). The prevalence of urinary incontinence in pregnancy among a multi-ethnic population resident in Norway. *Br. J. Obstet. Gynaecol.*, 119(11), 1354-1360.

[31] Fritel, X., Fauconnier, A., Bader, G., et al. (2010). Diagnosis and management of adult female stress urinary incontinence: guidelines for clinical practice from the French College of Gynaecologists and Obstetricians. *Eur. J. Obstet. Gynecol. Reprod. Biol.*, 151(1), 14-19.

[32] Di Stefano, M., Caserta, D., Marci, R., and Mosarini, M. (2000). Urinary incontinence in pregnancy and prevention of perineal complications of labor. *Minerva Ginecology*, 52, 307-311.

[33] Wijma, J., Weis Potters, A. E., Tinga, D. J., and Aarnoudse, J. G. (2008). The diagnostic strength of the 24-h pad test for self-reported symptoms of urinary incontinence in pregnancy and after childbirth. *Int. Urogynecol. J. Pelvic Floor Dysfunct.*, 19(4), 525-530.

[34] Cutner, A., Cardozo, L. D. and Benness, C. J. (1991). Assessment of urinary symptoms in early pregnancy. *Br. J. Obstet. Gynaecol.*, 98, 1283-1286.

[35] Thorp, J. M., Norton, P. A., Wall, L. L., Kuller, J. A., Eucker, B., and Wells, E. (1999). Urinary incontinence in pregnancy and the puerperium: a prospective study. *Am. J. Obstet. Gynecol.*, 181, 266-273.

[36] Van Kerrebroeck, P., Abrams, P., Chaikin, D., et al. (2002). The standardisation of terminology in nocturia: report from the

Standardisation Sub-committee of the International Continence Society. *Neurourol. Urodyn.*, 21(2), 179-183.

[37] Long, R. M., Giri, S. K. and Flood, H. D. (2008). Current concepts in female stress urinary incontinence. *Surgeon*, 6(6), 366-372.

[38] Hilde, G., Stær-Jensen, J., Ellström Engh, M., Brækken, I. H., and Bø, K. (2012). Continence and pelvic floor status in nulliparous women at midterm pregnancy. *Int. Urogynecol. J.*, 23(9), 1257-1263.

[39] Handa, V. L., Harris, T. A. and Ostergard, D. R. (1996). Protecting the pelvic floor: obstetric management to prevent incontinence and pelvic organ prolapse. *Obstet. Gynecol.*, 88, 470-478.

[40] Davis, K. and Kumar, D. (2003). Pelvic floor dysfunction: a conceptual framework for collaborative patient-centred care. *J. Adv. Nurs.*, 43(6), 555-568.

[41] Morkved, S., Bo, K., Schei, B., and Salvesen, K. A. (2003). Pelvic floor muscle training during pregnancy to prevent urinary incontinence: a single-blind randomized controlled trial. *Obstet. Gynecol.*, 101(2), 313-319.

[42] Morkved, S. and Bo, K. (2000). Effect of postpartum pelvic floor muscle training in prevention and treatment of urinary incontinence : a one-year follow up. *Br. J. Obstet. Gynaecol.*, 107(8), 1022-1028.

[43] Peyrat, L., Haillot, O., Bruyere, F., Boutin, J. M., Bertrand, P., and Lanson, Y. (2002). Prevalence and risk factors of urinary incontinence in young and middle-aged women. *BJU Int.*, 89, 61-66.

[44] Hermansen, I. L., O'Connell, B. and Gaskin, C. J. (2010). Are postpartum women in denmark being given helpful information about urinary incontinence and pelvic floor exercises? *J. Midwifery Womens Health*, 55(2), 171-174.

[45] Morkved, S., Salvesen, K. A., Bo, K., and Eik-Nes, S. (2004). Pelvic floor muscle strength and thickness in continent and incontinent nulliparous pregnant women. *Int. Urogynecol. J. Pelvic Floor Dysfunct.*, 15, 384-390.

[46] Hojberg, K. E., Salvig, J. D., Winslow, N. A., Lose, G., and Secher, N. J. (1999). Urinary incontinence: prevalence and risk factors at 16 weeks of gestation. *Br. J. Obstet. Gynaecol.*, 106, 842-850.

[47] MacLennan, A. H., Taylor, A. W., Wilson, D. H., and Wilson, D. (2000). The prevalence of pelvic floor disorder and their relationship to gender, age, parity and mode of delivery. *Br. J. Obstet. Gynaecol.*, 107, 1460-1470.

[48] Thom, D. H., Van den Eeden, S. K. and Brown, J. S. (1997). Evaluation of parturition and other reproductive variable as risk factors for incontinence later in life. *Obstet. Gynecol.*, 90, 983-989.

[49] Mikhail, M. S. and Anyaegbunam, A. (1995). Lower Urinary Tract Dysfunction in pregnancy: a review. *Obstet. Gynecol. Surv.*, 50(9), 675-683.

[50] Viktrup, L. (2002). The risk of urinary tract symptom five years after the first delivery. *Neurourol. Urodyn.*, 21(1), 2-29.

[51] Genadry, R. (2006). A urogynecologist's view ofthe pelvic floor effects of vaginal delivery/cesarean section for the urologist. *Curr. Urol. Rep.*, 7 (5), 376-383.

[52] Sangsawang, B. and Sangsawang, N. (2013). Stress urinary incontinence in pregnant women: a review of prevalence, pathophysiology, and treatment. *Int. Urogynecol. J.*, 24(6), 901-912.

[53] Wijma, J., Weis Potters, A. E., van der Mark, T. W., and Tinga, D. J. (2007). Aarnoudse JG.Displacement and recovery of the vesical neck position during pregnancy and after childbirth. *Neurourol. Urodyn.*, 26 (3), 372-376.

[54] Reed, H., Freeman, R. M., Waterfield, A., and Adekanmi, O. (2004). Prevalence of bladder neck mobility in asymptomatic non-pregnant nulliparous volunteers. *Br. J. Obstet. Gynaecol.*, 111(2), 172-175.

[55] Keane, D. P., Sims, T. J., Abrams, P., and Bailey, A. J., (1997). Analysis of collagen status in premenopausal nulliparous women with genuine stress incontinence. *Br. J. Obstet. Gynaecol.*, 104(9), 994-998.

[56] Dietz, H. P., Eldridge, A., Grace, M., and Clarke, B. (2004). Does pregnancy affect pelvic organ mobility? *Aust. N. Z. J. Obstet. Gynecol.*, 44, 517-520.

[57] King, J. K. and Freeman, R. M. (1998). Is antenatal bladder neck mobility a risk factor for postpartum stress urinary incontinence? *Br. J. Obstet. Gynaecol.*, 105, 1300-1307.

[58] Dickie, K. J., Shek, K. L. and Dietz, H. P. (2010). The relationship between urethral mobility and parity. *Br. J. Obstet. Gynaecol.*, 117(10), 1220-1224.

[59] Wijma, J., Weis Potters, A. E., de Wolf, B. T. H. M., Tinga, D. J., and Aarnoudse, J. G. (2001). Anatomical and functional changes in the lower urinary tract during pregnancy. *Br. J. Obstet. Gynaecol.*, 108, 726-732.

[60] Jundt, K., Scheer, I., Schiessl, B., Karl, K., Friese, K., and Peschers, U. M. (2010). Incontinence, bladder neck mobility, and sphincter ruptures in primiparous women. *Eur. J. Med. Res.*, 15(6), 246-252.

[61] Chaliha, C., Kalia, V., Stanton, S. L., Monga, A., and Sultan, A. H. (1999). Antenatal prediction of postpartum urinary and fecal incontinence. *Obstet. Gynecol.*, 94, 689-694.

[62] Freeman, R. M. (2013). Can we prevent childbirth-related pelvic floor dysfunction? *Br. J. Obstet. Gynaecol.*, 120(2), 137-140.

[63] Falconer, C., Ekman, G., Malmstrom, A., and Ulmsten, U. (1994). Decreased collagen synthesis in stress-incontinence women. *Obstet. Gynecol.*, 84, 583-586.

[64] Harvey, M. A., Johnston, S. L. and Davies, G. A. (2008). Mid-trimester serum relaxin concentrations and post-partum pelvic floor dysfunction. *Acta Obstet. Gynecol. Scand.*, 87(12), 1315-1321.

[65] Smith, A. L. and Wein, A. J. (2010). Estrogen replacement therapy for the treatment of postmenopausal genitourinary tract dysfunction. *Discov. Med.,* 10(55), 500-510.

[66] Hilton, P. and Dolan, L. M. (2004). Pathophysiology of urinary incontinence and pelvic organ prolapse. *Br. J. Obstet. Gynaecol.*, 111 (sup. 1), 5-9.

[67] Emmi, A. M., Skurnick, J., Goldsmith, L. T., et al. (1991). Ovarian control of pituitary hormone secretion in early human pregnancy. *J. Clin. Endocrinol. Metab.*, 72(6), 1359-1363.

[68] Kristiansson, P., Samuelsson, E., Schoultz, B., and Svardsudd, K. (2001). Reproductive hormones and stress urinary incontinence in pregnancy. *Acta Obstet. Gynecol. Scand.*, 80, 1125-1130.

[69] Harvey, M. A., Johnston, S. L. and Davies, G. A. (2004). Second trimester serum relaxin concentration are associated with pelvic organ prolapse following childbirth. *Paper presented at the 34th annual meeting of the International Continence Society*, Paris, French, August 25-27, 2004. Abstract retrieved September 27, 2005, from http://www. icsoffice.org/publications/ 2004/ PDF/0555PDF.

[70] Kristiansson, P., Svardsudd, K. and Schoultz, B. (1996). Serum relaxin, symphyseal pain, and back pain during pregnancy. *Am. J. Obstet. Gynecol.*, 175, 1342-1347.

[71] Petersen, L. K., Vogel, I., Agger, A. O., Westergard, J., Nils, M., and Uldbjerg, N. (1995). Variations in serum relaxin (hRLX-2) concentrations during human pregnany. *Acta Obstet. Gynecol. Scand.*, 74, 251-256.

[72] Chaliha, C. and Stanton, S. L. (2002). Urological problems in pregnancy. *BJU Int.*, 89, 469-476.

[73] Van Geelen, J. M., Lemmens, W. A., Eskes, T. K., and Martin, C. B. Jr. (1982). The urethral pressure profile in pregnancy and after delivery in healthy nulliparous women. *Am. J. Obstet. Gynecol.*, 144(6), 636-649.

[74] Suckling, J., Lethaby, A. and Kennedy, R. (2006). Local oestrogen for vaginal atrophy in postmenopausal women. *Cochrane Database Syst. Rev.*, (4), CD001500.

[75] Robinson, D. and Carozo, L. (2004). Oestrogens and the lower urinary tract. *Br. J. Obstet. Gynaecol.*, 111(sup. 1), 10-14.

[76] Swift, S. E. and Ostergard, D. R. (1993). Effects of progesterone on the urinary tract. *Int. Urogynecol. J.*, 4(4), 232-236.

[77] Tincello, D. G., Teare, J. and Fraser, W. D. (2003). Second trimester concentration of relaxin and pregnancy related incontinence. *Eur. J. Obstet. Gynecol. Reprod. Biol.*, 106, 237-238.

[78] Chaliha, C., Bland, J. M., Monga, A., Stanton, S. L., and Sultan, A. H. (2000). Pregnancy and derivery: a urodynamic viewpoint. *Br. J. Obstet. Gynaecol.*, 107, 1354-1359.

[79] Hvidman, L., Foldspang, A., Mommsen, S., and Nielsen, J. B. (2002). Correlates of urinary incontinence in pregnancy. *Int. Urogynecol. J. Pelvic Floor Dysfunct.*, 13, 278-283.

[80] Allahdin, S. and Kambhampati, L. (2012). Stress urinary incontinence in continent primigravidas. *J. Obstet. Gynaecol.*, 32(1), 2-5.

[81] Groutz, A., Helpman, L., Gold, R., Pauzner, D., Lessing, J. B., and Gordon, D. (2007). First vaginal delivery at an older age: Does it carry an extra risk for the development of stress urinary incontinence? *Neurourol. Urodyn.*, 26(6), 779-782.

[82] Glazener, C. M., Herbison, G. P., MacArthur, C., et al. (2006). New postnatal urinary incontinence: obstetric and other risk factors in primiparae. *Br. J. Obstet. Gynaecol.*, 113(2), 208-217.

[83] Dietz, H. P. and Wilson, P. D. (2005). Childbirth and pelvic floor trauma. *Best Pract. Res. Clin. Obstet. Gynaecol.*, 19, 913-924.

[84] Rud, T. (1980). Urethral pressure profile in continent women from childhood to old age. *Acta Obstet. Gynecol. Scand.*, 59, 331-335.

[85] Pandit, M., DeLancey, J. O., Ashton-Miller, J. A., Iyengar, J., Blaivas, M., and Perucchini, D. (2000). Quantification of intramuscular nerves within the female striated urogenital sphincter muscle. *Obstet. Gynecol.*, 95, 797-800.

[86] Perucchini, D., DeLancey, J. O., Ashton-Miller, J. A., Peschers, U., and Kataria, T. (2002). Age effects on urethral striated muscle. I. Changes in

number and diameter of striated muscle fibers in the ventral urethra. *Am. J. Obstet. Gynecol.*, 186, 351-355.

[87] Hijaz, A., Sadeghi, Z., Byrne, L., Hou, J. C., and Daneshgari, F. (2012). Advanced maternal age as a risk factor for stress urinary incontinence: a review of the literature. *Int. Urogynecol. J.*, 23, 395-401.

[88] Trowbridge, E. R., Wei, J. T., Fenner, D. E., Ashton-Miller, J. A., and Delancey, J. O. (2007). Effects of aging on lower urinary tract and pelvic floor function in nulliparous women. *Obstet. Gynecol.*, 109(3), 715-720.

[89] Lewicky-Gaupp, C., Cao, D. C. and Culbertson, S. (2008). Urinary and anal incontinence in African American teenaged gravidas during pregnancy and the puerperium. *J. Pediatr. Adolesc. Gynecol.*, 21(1), 21-26.

[90] Arrue, M., Ibañez, L., Paredes, J., et al. (2010). Stress urinary incontinence six months after first vaginal delivery. *Eur. J. Obstet. Gynecol. Reprod. Biol.*, 150(2), 210-214.

[91] Meyer, S., Schreyer, A., Grandi, P., and Hohlfeld, P. (1998). The effect of birth on urinary incontinence mechanisms and other pelvic-floor characteristics. *Obstet. Gynecol.*, 92(4), 613-618.

[92] Marshall, K., Thompson, K. A., Walsh, D. M., and Baxter, G. D. (1998). Incidence of urinary incontinence and constipation during pregnancy and postpartum: survey of current findings at the Rotunda Lying-in Hospital. *Br. J. Obstet. Gynaecol.*, 105, 400-402.

[93] Meyer, S., Bachelard, O. and De Grandi, P. (1998). Do bladder neck mobility and urethral sphincter function differ during pregnancy compared with during the non-pregnant state? *Int. Urogynecol. J. Pelvic Floor Dysfunct.*, 9(6), 397-404.

[94] Zhu, L., Bian, X. M., Long, Y., and Lang, J. H. (2008). Role of different childbirth strategies on pelvic organ prolapse and stress urinary incontinence: a prospective study. *Chin. Med. J.*, 121(3), 213-215.

[95] Chaliha, C. (2009). Postpartum pelvic floor trauma. *Curr. Opin. Obstet. Gynecol.*, 21(6), 474-479.

[96] Herbruck, L. F. (2008). The impact of childbirth on the pelvic floor. *Urol. Nurs.*, 28(3),173-184.

[97] Tunn, R., Goldammer, K., Neymeyer, J., Gauruder-Burmester, A., Hamm, B., and Beyersdorff, D. (2006). MRI morphology of the levator ani muscle, endopelvic fascia, and urethra in women with stress urinary incontinence. *Eur. J. Obstet. Gynecol. Reprod. Biol.*, 126(2), 239-245.

[98] Torrisi, G., Minini, G., Bernasconi, F., et al. (2012). A prospective study of pelvic floor dysfunctions related to delivery. *Eur. J. Obstet. Gynecol. Reprod. Biol.*, 160(1), 110-115.
[99] Leijonhufvud, A., Lundholm, C., Cnattingius, S., Granath, F., Andolf, E., and Altman, D. (2011). Risks of stress urinary incontinence and pelvic organ prolapse surgery in relation to mode of childbirth. *Am. J. Obstet. Gynecol.*, 204(1), 70.e1-7.
[100] Yang, X., Zhang, H. X., Yu, H. Y., Gao, X. L., Yang, H. X., and Dong, Y. (2010). The prevalence of fecal incontinence and urinary incontinence in primiparous postpartum Chinese women. *Eur. J. Obstet. Gynecol. Reprod. Biol.*, 152(2), 214-217.
[101] Goldberg, R. P., Abramov, Y., Botros, S., et al. (2005). Delivery mode is a major environmental determinant of stress urinary incontinence: results of the Evanston-Northwestern Twin Sisters Study. *Am. J. Obstet. Gynecol.*, 193(6), 2149-2153.
[102] Wesnes, S. L., Hunskaar, S., Bo, K., and Rortveit, G. (2009). The effect of urinary incontinence status during pregnancy and delivery mode on incontinence postpartum. A cohort study. *Br. J. Obstet. Gynaecol.*, 116 (5), 700-707.
[103] Arya, L. A., Jackson, N. D., Myers, D. L., and Verma, A. (2001). Risk of new-onset urinary incontinence after forceps and vacuum delivery in primiparous women. *Am. J. Obstet. Gynecol.*, 185(6), 1318-1324.
[104] Van Kessel, K., Reed, S., Newton, K., Meier, A., and Lentz, G. (2001). The second stage of labor and stress urinary incontinence. *Am. J. Obstet. Gynecol.*, 184(7),1571-1575.
[105] Hantoushzadeh, S., Javadian, P., Shariat, M., Salmanian, B., Ghazizadeh, S., and Aghssa, M. (2011). Stress urinary incontinence: pre-pregnancy history and effects of mode of delivery on its postpartum persistency. *Int. Urogynecol. J.*, 22(6), 651-655.
[106] Panayi, D. C. and Khullar, V. (2009). Urogynaecological problems in pregnancy and postpartum sequelae. *Curr. Opin. Obstet. Gynecol.*, 21 (1), 97-100.
[107] Eftekhar, T., Hajibaratali, B., Ramezanzadeh, F., and Shariat, M. (2006). Postpartum evaluation of stress urinary incontinence among primiparas. *Int. J. Gynaecol. Obstet.*, 94(2), 114-118.
[108] Boyles, S. H., Li, H., Mori, T., Osterweil, P., and Guise, J. M. (2009). Effect of mode of delivery on the incidence of urinary incontinence in primiparous women. *Obstet. Gynecol.*, 113(1), 134-141.

[109] Fritel, X., Ringa, V., Quiboeuf, E., and Fauconnier, A. (2012). Female urinary incontinence, from pregnancy to menopause: a review of epidemiological and pathophysiological findings. *Acta Obstet. Gynecol. Scand.*, 91(8), 901-910.

[110] Altman, D., Ekström, A., Forsgren, C., Nordenstam, J., and Zetterström, J. (2007). Symptoms of anal and urinary incontinence following cesarean section or spontaneous vaginal delivery. *Am. J. Obstet. Gynecol.*, 197(5), 512.e1-7.

[111] Chou, P. L., Chen, F. P. and Teng, L. F. (2005). Factors associated with urinary stress incontinence in primiparas. *Taiwan J. Obstet. Gynecol.*, 44, 42-47.

[112] Burgio, K. L., Zyczynski, H., Locher, J. L., Richter, H. E., Redden, D. T., and Wright, K. C. (2003). Urinary incontinence in the 12-month postpartum period. *Obstet. Gynecol.*, 102, 1291-1298.

[113] Wilson, P. D., Herbison, R. M. and Herbison, G. P. (1996). Obstetric practice and the prevalence of Urinary Incontinence three months after delivery. *Br. J. Obstet. Gynaecol.*, 103(1), 154-161.

[114] Pregazzi, R., Sartore, A., Troiano, L., et al. (2002). Postpartum Urinary symptoms: prevalence and risk factors. *Obstet. Gynecol.*, 103(2),179-182.

[115] Greer, W. J., Richter, H. E., Bartolucci, A. A., and Burgio, K. L. (2008). Obesity and pelvic floor disorders: a systematic review. *Obstet. Gynecol.*, 112(2 Pt 1), 341-349.

[116] Bump, R. C., Sugerman, H., Fantl, J. A., and McClish, D. M. (1992). Obesity and lower urinary tract function in women: effect of surgically induced weight loss. *Am. J. Obstet. Gynecol.*, 166, 392-399.

[117] Ebbesen, M. H., Hannestad, Y. S., Midthjell, K., and Hunskaar, S. (2007). Diabetes and urinary incontinence - prevalence data from Norway. *Acta Obstet. Gynecol. Scand.*, 86(10), 1256-1262.

[118] Hannestad, Y. S., Rortveit, G., Daltveit, A. K., and Hunskaar, S. (2003). Are smoking and other lifestyle factors associated with female urinary incontinence? The Norwegian EPINCONT Study. *Br. J. Obstet. Gynaecol.*, 110(3), 247-254.

[119] Danforth, K. N., Townsend, M. K., Lifford, K., Curhan, G. C., Resnick, N. M., and Grodstein, F. (2006). Risk factors for urinary incontinence among middle-aged women. *Am. J. Obstet. Gynecol.*, 194(2), 339-345.

[120] Bump, R. C. and McClish, D. M. (1994). Cigarette smoking and pure genuine stress incontinence of urine: a comparison of risk factors and

determinants between smokers and nonsmokers. *Am. J. Obstet. Gynecol.*, 170, 579-582.

[121] Bradley, C. S., Kennedy, C. M., Turcea, A. M., Rao, S. S., and Nygaard, I. E. (2007). Constipation in pregnancy: prevalence, symptoms, and risk factors. *Obstet. Gynecol.*, 110(6), 1351-1357.

[122] Bonapace, E. S. Jr. and Fisher, R. S. (1998). Constipation and diarrhea in pregnancy. *Gastroenterol. Clin. North Am.*, 27, 197-211.

[123] Van Brummen, H. J., Bruinse, H. W., van de Pol, G., Heintz, A. P., and van der Vaart, C. H. (2006). Defecatory symptoms during and after the first pregnancy: prevalences and associated factors. *Int. Urogynecol. J. Pelvic Floor Dysfunct.*, 17, 224-230.

[124] Penn, C., Lekan-Rutledge, D., Joers, A. M., Stolley, J. M., and Amhof, N. V. (1996). Assessment of urinary incontinence. *J. Gerontol. Nurs.*, 22 (1), 8-19.

[125] Amselem, C., Puigdollers, A., Azpiroz, F., et al. (2010). Constipation: a potential cause of pelvic floor damage? *Neurogastroenterol. Motil.*, 22 (2), 150-153.

[126] Fritel, X., Fauconnier, A., Levet, C., and Bénifla, J. L. (2004). Stress urinary incontinence 4 years after the first delivery: a retrospective cohort survey. *Acta Obstet. Gynecol. Scand.*, 83(10), 941-945.

[127] Landon, C. R., Crofts, C. E., Smith, A. R. B., and Trowbridge, E. A. (1990). Mechanical properties of fascia during pregnancy: a possible factor in the development of stress incontinence of urine. *Contemp. Rev. Obstet. Gynaecol.*, 2, 40-46.

[128] Stainton, M. C., Strahle, A. and Fethney, J. (2005). Leaking urine prior to pregnancy: a risk factor for postnatal incontinence. *Aust. N. Z. J. Obstet. Gynaecol.*, 45(4), 295-299.

[129] Melville, J. L., Katon, W., Delaney, K., and Newton, K. (2005). Urinary incontinence in US women: a population-based study. *Arch. Intern. Med.*, 165(5), 537-542.

[130] Saydah, S. H., Chandra, A. and Eberhardt, M. S. (2005). Pregnancy experience among women with and without gestational diabetes in the US, 1995 National survey of family growth. *Diabetes Care*, 28(5), 1035-1040.

[131] Brown, J. S., Nyberg, L. M., Kusek, J. W., Burgio, K. L., and Diokno, A. C. (2003). Proceedings of the national institute of diabetes and digestive and kidney diseases international symposium on epidemiologic issues in urinary incontinence in women. *Am. J. Obstet. Gynecol.*, 188 (6), S77-S88.

[132] Kim, C., McEwen, L. N., Sarma, A. V., Piette, J. D., and Herman, W. H. (2008). Stress urinary incontinence in women with a history of gestational diabetes mellitus. *J. Womens Health*, 17(5), 783-792.
[133] Chuang, C. M., Lin, I. F., Horng, H. C., Hsiao, Y. H., Shyu, I. L., and Chou, P. (2012). The impact of gestational diabetes mellitus on postpartum urinary incontinence: a longitudinal cohort study on singleton pregnancies. *Br. J. Obstet. Gynecol.*, 119, 1334-1343.
[134] Lee, A. H. and Hirayama, F. (2012). Alcohol consumption and female urinary incontinence: a community-based study in Japan. *Int. J. Urol.*, 19(2), 143-148.
[135] Bryant, C. M., Dowell, C. J. and Fairbrother, G. (2002). Caffeine reduction education to improve urinary symptoms. *Br. J. Nurs.*, 11(8), 560-565.
[136] Gleason, J. L., Richter, H. E., Redden, D. T., Goode, P. S., Burgio, K. L., and Markland, A. D. (2013). Caffeine and urinary incontinence in US women. *Int. Urogynecol. J.*, 24(2), 295-302.
[137] Sangsawang, B. (2014). Risk factors for the development of stress urinary incontinence during pregnancy in primigravidae: a review of the literature. *Eur. J. Obstet. Gynecol. Reprod. Biol.*, 178C, 27-34.
[138] Salvatore, S., Khullar, V., Cardozo, L., Anders, K., Zocchi, G., and Soligo, M. (2001). Evaluating ambulatory urodynamics: a prospective study in asymptomatic women. *Br. J. Obstet. Gynecol.*, 108(1), 107-111.
[139] Pantazis, K. and Freeman, R. M. (2006). Investigation and treatment of urinary incontinence. *Curr. Obstet. Gynecol.*, 16, 344-352.
[140] Smith, C. A. and Witherow, R. O. (2000). The assessment of female pelvic floor dysfunction. *BJU Int.*, 85(5), 579-587.
[141] Kelleher, C. J., Cardozo, L. D., Khullar, V., and Salvatore, S. (1997). A new questionnaire to assess the quality of life of urinary incontinence women. *Br. J. Obstet. Gynecol.*, 104, 1374-1379.
[142] Shumaker, S. A., Wyman, J. F., Uebersax, J. S., McClish, D., and Fantl, J. A. (1994). Health-related quality of life measures for women with urinary incontinence: the Incontinence Impact Questionnaire and the Urogenital Distress Inventory. Continence Program in Women (CPW) Research Group. *Qual. Life Res.*, 3(5), 291-306.
[143] Kocaöz, S., Talas, M. S. and Atabekoğlu, C. S. (2010). Urinary incontinence in pregnant women and their quality of life. *J. Clin. Nurs.*, 19(23-24), 3314-3323.
[144] Norton, P. A. (1990). Prevalence and social impact of urinary incontinence in women. *Clin. Obstet. Gynecol.*, 33(2), 295-297.

[145] Temml, C., Haidinger, G., Schmidbauer, J., Schatzl, G., and Madersbacher, S. (2000). Urinary incontinence in both sexes: prevalence rates and impact on quality of life and sexual life. *Neurourol. Urodyn.*, 19(3), 259-271.

[146] Hatem, M., Fraser, W. and Lepire, E. (2005). Postpartum urinary and anal incontinence: a population-based study of quality of life of primiparous women in Quebec. *J. Obstet. Gynaecol. Can.*, 27(7), 682-688.

[147] Mascarenhas, T., Coelho, R., Oliveira, M., and Patricio, B. (2003). Impact of urinary incontinence on quality of life during pregnancy and after childbirth. *Paper presented at the 33th annual meeting of the International Continence Society*, Florence, Italy, October 9, 2003.

[148] Dolan, L. M., Walsh, D., Hamilton, S., Marshall, K., Thompson, K., and Ashe, R. G. (2004). A study of quality of life in primigravidae with urinary incontinence. *Int. Urogynecol. J. Pelvic Floor Dysfunct.*, 15, 160-164.

[149] Van de Pol, G. G., Van Brummen, H. J., Bruinse, H. W., Heintz, A. P., and van der Vaart, C. H. (2007). Is there an association between depressive and urinary symptoms during and after pregnancy? *Int. Urogynecol. J. Pelvic Floor Dysfunct.*, 18, 1409-1415.

[150] Adaji, S. E., Shittu, O. S., Bature, S. B., Nasir, S., and Olatunji, O. (2010). Suffering in silence: pregnant women's experience of urinary incontinence in Zaria, Nigeria. *Eur. J. Obstet. Gynecol. Reprod. Biol.*, 150(1), 19-23.

[151] Marecki, M. and Seo, J. Y. (2010). Perinatal urinary and fecal incontinence: suffering in silence. *J. Perinat. Neonatal. Nurs.*, 24(4), 330-340.

[152] Newman, D. K. (2001). Conservative management of urinary incontinence in women. *Prim. Care Update Ob. Gyns.*, 8(4), 153-162.

[153] Hvidman, L., Foldspang, A., Mommsen, S., and Nielsen, J. B. (2003). Postpartum urinary incontinence. *Acta Obstet. Gynecol. Scand.*, 82, 556-563.

[154] Dimpl, T. H., Hesse, U. and Schuessler, B. (1992). Incidence and cause of postpartum urinary stress incontinence. *Eur. J. Obstet. Gynecol. Reprod. Biol.*, 43(1), 29-33.

[155] Foldspang, A., Hvidman, L., Mommsen, S., and Nielsen, J. B. (2004). Risk of postpartum Urinary Incontinence associated with pregnancy and mode of delivery. *Acta Obstet. Gynecol. Scand.*, 83, 923-927.

[156] Goldberg, R. P., Know, C., Gandhi, S., Atkuru, L. V., Sorensen, M., and Sand, P. K. (2003). Urinary incontinence among mother of multiples: The protective effect of cesarean delivery. *Am. J. Obstet. Gynecol.*, 188, 1447-1453.

[157] Glazener, C. M. A., Herbison, G. P., Wilson, P. D., et al. (2001). Conservative management of persistent postnatal urinary and faecal incontinence: randomized controlled trial. *BMJ*, 323, 593-596.

[158] Dumoulin, C., Lemieux, M. C., Bourbonnais, D., Gravel, D., Bravo, G., and Morin, M. (2004). Physiotherapy for persistent postnatal stress urinary incontinence: a randomized controlled trial. *Obstet. Gynecol.*, 104, 504-510.

[159] Reilly, E. T. C., Freeman, R. M., Waterfield, M. R., Waterfield, A. E., Steggles, P., and Pedlar, F. (2002). Prevention of postpartum stress incontinence in primigravidae with increased bladder neck mobility: a randomised controlled trial of antenatal pelvic floor exercise. *Br. J. Obstet. Gynecol.*, 109(1), 68-76.

[160] Herzog, A. R., Diokno, A. C., Brown, M. B., Fultz, N. H., and Goldstein, N. E. (1994). Urinary incontinence as a risk factor for mortality. *J. Am. Geriatr. Soc.*, 42, 264-268.

[161] Sampselle, C. M., Miller, J. M., Mims, B. L., Delancey, J. O. L., Ashton-Miller, J. A., and Antonakos, C. L. (1998). Effect of pelvic muscle exercise on transient incontinence during pregnancy and after birth. *Obstet. Gynecol.*, 91(3), 406-412.

[162] Bo, K. (1994). Reproducibility of instruments designed to measure subjective evaluation of female stress urinary incontinence. *Scand. J. Urol. Nephrol.*, 28, 97-100.

[163] Frazer, M. I., Heylen, B. T. and Sutherst, J. R. (1989). The severity of urinary incontinence in women: Comparison of subjective and objective test. *Br. J. Urol.*, 63, 14-15.

[164] Stach-Lempinen, B., Kujansuu, E., Laippala, P., and Metsanoja, R. (2001). Visual analogue scale, Urinary incontinence severity score and 15 D-Psychometric testing of three different health-related quality of life instrument for urinary incontinence women. *Scand. J. Urol. Nephrol.*, 35, 476-483.

[165] Seeger, D., Truong, S. T. and Kimmig, R. (2006). Spontaneous delivery following tension-free vaginal tape procedure. *Int. Urogynecol. J. Pelvic Floor Dysfunct.*, 17(6), 676-678.

[166] Groenen, R., Vos, M. C., Willekes, C., and Vervest, H. A. (2008). Pregnancy and delivery after mid-urethral sling procedures for stress

urinary incontinence: case reports and a review of literature. *Int. Urogynecol. J. Pelvic Floor Dysfunct.*, 19(3), 441-448.

[167] Neumann, P. B., Grimmer, K. A., Grant, R. E., and Gill, V. A. (2005). The costs and benefits of physiotherapy as first-line treatment for female stress urinary incontinence. *Aust. N. Z. J. Public Health,* 29(5), 416-421.

[168] Ferguson, K. L., McKey, P. L., Bishop, K. R., Verheul, J. B., and Dougherty, M. C. (1990). Stress urinary incontinence: Effect of pelvic muscle exercise. *Obstet. Gynecol.*, 75(4), 671-675.

[169] Kolcaba, K. and Dowd, T. (2000). Kegel Exercises: Strengthening the weak pelvic floor muscle that cause urinary incontinence. *Am. J. Nurs.,* 100(11), 59.

[170] Wagg, A. and Bunn, F. (2007). Unassisted pelvic floor exercises for postnatal women: a systematic review. *J. Adv. Nurs.*, 58(5), 407-417.

[171] Boyle, R., Hay-Smith, E. J., Cody, J. D., and Mørkved, S. (2012). Pelvic floor muscle training for prevention and treatment of urinary and faecal incontinence in antenatal and postnatal women. *Cochrane Database Syst. Rev.*, 10: CD007471.

[172] Hay-Smith, E. J. C., Herderschee, R., Dumoulin, C., and Herbison, G. P. (2011). Comparisons of approaches to pelvic floor muscle train-ing for urinary incontinence in women. *Cochrane Database Syst. Rev.*, 12, CD 009508.

[173] Di Benedetto, P., Coidessa, A. and Floris, S. (2008). Rationale of pelvic floor muscles training in women with urinary incontinence. *Minerva Ginecol.*, 60(6), 529-541.

[174] Kegel, N. (1948). Progressive resistance exercise in the functional retroration of the perineal muscle. *Am. J. Obstet. Gynecol.*, 56, 238-248.

[175] Bump, R. C., Hurt, W. G., Fantl, J. A., and Wyman, J. F. (1991). Assessment of kegel pelvic muscle exercise performance after brief verbal instruction. *Am. J. Obstet. Gynecol.*, 165, 322-329.

[176] Newman, D. K. and Smith, D. A. (1992). Pelvic muscle reeducation as a nursing treatment for incontinence. *Urol. Nurs.*, 12(1), 9-15.

[177] Beckman, N. J. (1995). An overview of urinary incontinence in adults: Assessment and behavioral intervention. *Clin. Nurse Spec.*, 9(5), 241-247.

[178] DiNubile, N. A. (1991). Strength training. *Clin. Sports Med.*, 10(1), 33-62.

[179] American College of Sports Medicine [ACSM]. (1991). *Guideline for exercise testing and prescription.* (4th ed.). Philadelphia: Lea and Febiger.

[180] Andersen, J. T., Blaivas, J. G., Cardozo, L., and Thuroff, J. (1992). ICS 7th Report on the standardisation of terminology of lower urinary tract function lower urinary tract rehabilitation techniques. *Neurourol. Urodyn.*, 11, 593-603.

[181] Fantl, J. A., Newman, D. K., Colling, J., et al. (1996). *Urinary incontinence in adult: Acute and chronic management* (Clinical practice guideline, No. 2, 1996 Update, US Department of Health and Human Services. Public Health Service, Agency for Health Care Policy and Research. AHCPR Publication No. 96-0682. March 1996.) Retrieved July 20, 2005, from http://www. ncbi.nlm.nih.gov/books/bv.fcgi? rid= hstat6. chapter. 32554.

[182 Johnson, S. T. (2000). From incontinence to confidence. *Am. J. Nurs.*, 100(2), 69-75.

[183] National Institutes of Health Consensus Development Conference. (1990). Urinary incontinence in adult. *J. Am. Geriatr. Soc.*, 38, 265-272.

[184] Holroy-Ledue, J. M. and Straus, S. E. (2004). Management of Urinary Incontinence in Women. *JAMA*, 291(8), 996-999.

[185] Sangsawang, B. (2007). Effect of pelvic floor muscle exercise program on severity of stress urinary incontinence among pregnant women [*Master' s thesis*]. Mahidol University, Thailand: Bangkok.

[186] Bø, K. (2004). Pelvic floor muscle training is effective in treatment of female stress urinary incontinence, but how does it work? *Int. Urogynecol. J. Pelvic Floor Dysfunct.*, 15(2), 76-84.

[187] Jozwik, M. and Jozwik, M. (1998). The physiological basis of pelvic floor exercises in the treatment of stress urinary incontinence. *Br. J. Obstet. Gynecol.*, 105, 1046-1051.

[188] Gosling, J. A., Dixon, J. S., Critchley, H. O., and Thompson, S. A. (1981). A comparative study of the human external sphincter and periurethral levator ani muscles. *Br. J. Urol.*, 53(1), 35-41.

[189] Kegel A. H. (1952). Stress incontinence and genital relaxation; a nonsurgical method of increasing the tone of sphincters and their supporting structures. *Ciba Clin. Symp.*, 4(2), 35-51.

[190] Bø, K., Kvarstein, B., Hagen, R., and Larsen, S. (1990). Pelvic floormuscle exercise for the treatment of female stress urinary incontinence: I. Reliability of vaginal pressure measurements of pelvic floor muscle strength. *Neurourol. Urodyn.*, 9, 471-477.

[191] Chiarelli, P., Murphy, B. and Cockburn, J. (2003). Women's knowledge, practises, and intentions regarding correct pelvic floor exercises. *Neurourol. Urodyn.*, 22(3), 246-249.

[192] Wilson, P. D. and Herbison, G. P. (1998). A randomized controlled trial of pelvic floor muscle exercises to treat postnatal urinary incontinence. *Int. Urogynecol. J. Pelvic Floor Dysfunct.*, 9(5), 257-264.

[193] Henderson, J. W., Wang, S., Egger, M. J., Masters, M., and Nygaard, I. (2013). Can women correctly contract their pelvic floor muscles without formal instruction? *Female Pelvic Med. Reconstr. Surg.*, 19(1), 8-12.

[194] Chiarelli, P. and Cockburn, J. (1999). The development of a physiotherapy continence promotion program using a customer focus. *Aust. J. Physiother.*, 45(2), 111-119.

[195] Sampselle, C. M. (2000). Behavioral intervention for urinary incontinence in women: evidence for practice. *J. Midwifery Womens Health*, 45(2), 94-103.

[196] Sampselle, C. M., Brink, C. A. and Wells, T. J. (1989). Digital measurement of pelvic muscle strength in childbearing women. *Nurs. Res.*, 38(3), 134-138.

[197] Pearson, B. D. and Kelber, S. (1996). Urinary incontinence: Treatment, intervention, and outcome. *Clin. Nurse Spec.*, 10(4), 177-182.

[198] Sampselle, C. M. (1990). Changes in pelvic floor muscle strength associated with childbirth. *J. Obstet. Gynecol. Neonatal Nurs.*, 19(5), 371-377.

[199] Cammu, H. and Nylen, M. V. (1995). Pelvic floor muscle exercise: 5 years later. *Urology,* 45(1), 113-117.

[200] Hahn, I., Milsom, I., Fall, M., and Ekelund, P. (1993). Long-term results of pelvic floor training in female stress urinary incontinence. *Br. J. Urol.*, 72, 421-427.

[201] Berghmans, L. C. M., Hendriks, H. J. M., Bo, K., Hay-Smith, E. J., de Bie, R. A., and van Waalwijk van Doorn, E. S. C. (1998). Conservative treatment of stress urinary incontinence in women: a systematic review of randomized clinical trials. *Br. J. Urol.*, 82, 181-191.

[202] Dumoulin, C., Glazener, C. and Jenkinson, D. (2011). Determining the optimal pelvic floor muscle training regimen for women with stress urinary incontinence. *Neurourol. Urodyn.*, 30(5), 746-753.

[203] Mason, L., Glenn, S., Walton, I., and Hughes, C. (2001). The instruction in pelvic floor exercise provided to women during pregnancy or following delivery. *Midwifery,* 17, 55-64.

[204] Bo, K., Hagen, R. H., Kvarstein, B., Jorgensen, J., and Larson, S. (1990). Pelvic floor muscle exercise for the treatment of female stress urinary incontinence. III. Effect of two different degrees of pelvic floor muscle exercise. *Neurourol. Urodyn.*, 9, 489-502.

[205] Griffin, C., Dougherty, M. C. and Yarandi, H. (1994). Pelvic muscles during rest: responses to pelvic muscle exercise. *Nurs. Res.*, 43(3), 164-167.

[206] Dinc, A., Kizilkaya Beji, N. and Yalcin, O. (2009). Effect of pelvic floor muscle exercises in the treatment of urinary incontinence during pregnancy and the postpartum period. *Int. Urogynecol. J. Pelvic Floor Dysfunct.*, 20(10), 1223-1231.

[207] Kocaöz, S., Eroğlu, K. and Sivaslıoğlu, A. A. (2013). Role of pelvic floor muscle exercises in the prevention of stress urinary incontinence during pregnancy and the postpartum period. *Gynecol. Obstet. Invest.*, 75(1), 34-40.

[208] Sangsawang, B. and Serisathien, Y. (2011). Effect of pelvic floor muscle exercise programme on stress urinary incontinence among pregnant women. *J. Adv. Nurs.*, 68(9), 1997-2007.

[209] Ko, P. C., Liang, C. C., Chang, S. D., Lee, J. T., Chao, A. S., and Cheng, P. J. (2011). A randomized controlled trial of antenatal pelvic floor exercises to prevent and treat urinary incontinence. *Int. Urogynecol. J.*, 22(1), 17-22.

[210] Stafne, S., Salvesen, K., Romundstad, P., Torjusen, I., and Mørkved, S. (2012). Does regular exercise including pelvic floor muscle training prevent urinary and anal incontinence during pregnancy? A randomised controlled trial. *Br. J. Obstet. Gynaecol.*, 119(10), 1270-1280.

[211] Pelaez, M., Gonzalez-Cerron, S., Montejo, R., and Barakat, R. (2014). Pelvic floor muscle training included in a pregnancy exercise program is effective in primary prevention of urinary incontinence: a randomized controlled trial. *Neurourol. Urodyn.*, 33(1), 67-71.

[212] Mason, L., Roe, B., Wong, H., Davies, J., and Bamber, J. (2010). The role of antenatal pelvic floor muscle exercises in prevention of postpartum stress incontinence: a randomised controlled trial. *J. Clin. Nurs.*, 19(19-20), 2777-2786.

[213] Fine, P., Burgio, K., Borello-France, D., et al. (2007). Teaching and practicing of pelvic floor muscle exercises in primiparous women during pregnancy and the postpartum period. *Am. J. Obstet. Gynecol.*, 197: 107.e1-107.e5.

[214] Bø, K. and Talseth, T. (1996). Long-term effect of pelvic floor muscle exercise 5 years after cessation of organized training. *Obstet. Gynecol.*, 87(2), 261-265.

[215] Bø, K., Kvarstein, B. and Nygaard, I. (2005). Lower urinary tract symptoms and pelvic floor muscle exercise adherence after 15 years. *Obstet. Gynecol.*, 105(5 Pt 1), 999-1005.

[216] Alewijnse, D., Mesters, I., Metsemakers, J., and van den Borne, B. (2003). Predictors of long-term adherence to pelvic floor muscle exercise therapy among women with urinary incontinence. *Health Educ. Res.*, 18(5), 511-524.

[217] Holley, R. L., Varner, R. E., Kerns, D. J., and Mestecky, P. J. (1995). Long-term failure of pelvic floor musculature exercises in treatment of genuine stress incontinence. *South Med. J.*, 88(5), 547-549.

[218] Milne, J. L. and Moore, K. N. (2006). Factors impacting self-care for urinary incontinence. *Urol. Nurs.*, 26(1), 41-51.

[219] Hay-Smith, E. J. C., Ryan, K. and Dean, S. (2007). The silent, private exercise: experiences of pelvic floor muscle training in a sample of women with stress urinary incontinence. *Physiotherapy*, 93, 53-61.

[220] Kincade, J. E., Johnson, T. M., Ashford-Works, C., Clarke, M. K., and Busby-Whitehead, J. (1999). A Pilot Study to Determine Reasons for Patient Withdrawal From a Pelvic Muscle Rehabilitation Program for Urinary Incontinence. *J. Appl. Gerontol.*, 18, 379-396.

[221] Ashworth, P. D. and Hagan, M. T. (1993). Some Social Consequences of Non-compliance with Pelvic Floor Exercises. *Physiotherapy*, 79(7), 465-471.

[222] Borello-France, D., Burgio, K. L., Goode, P. S., et al. (2013). Adherence to behavioral interventions for stress incontinence: rates, barriers, and predictors. *Phys. Ther.*, 93(6), 757-773.

[223] Bishop, K. R., Dougherty, M., Mooney, R., Gimotty, P., and Williams, B. (1992). Effect of age, parity and adherence on pelvic muscle respond to exercise. *J. Obstet. Gynecol. Neonatal Nurs.*, 21(5), 371-377.

[224] Bø, K., Owe, K. M. and Nystad, W. (2007). Which women do pelvic floor muscle exercises six months' postpartum? *Am. J. Obstet. Gynecol.*, 197(1), 49.e1-5.

[225] Elia, G. and Bergman, A. (1993). Pelvic muscle exercises: when do they work? *Obstet. Gynecol.*, 81(2), 283-286.

[226] Cammu, H., Van Nylen, M., Blockeel, C., Kaufman, L., and Amy, J. J. (2004). Who will benefit from pelvic floor muscle training for stress urinary incontinence? *Am. J. Obstet. Gynecol.*, 191(4), 1152-1157.

[227] Burgio, K. L., Goode, P. S., Locher, J. L., et al. (2003). Predictors of outcome in the behavioral treatment of urinary incontinence in women. *Obstet. Gynecol.*, 102(5 Pt 1), 940-947.

[228] Chen, S. Y. and Tzeng, Y. L. (2009). Path analysis for adherence to pelvic floor muscle exercise among women with urinary incontinence. *J. Nurs. Res.*, 17(2), 83-92.

[229] Mason, L., Glenn, S., Walton, I., and Hughes, C. (2001). Do Women Practise Pelvic Floor Exercises during Pregnancy or following Delivery? *Physiotherapy*, 87(12), 662-670.

[230] Alewijnse, D., Mesters, I., Metsemakers, J., Ad-riaans, J., and van den Borne, B. (2001). Predictors of inten-tion to adhere to physiotherapy among women with urinary incontinence. *Health Ed. Res.*, 16, 173-186.

[231] Hung, H. C., Chih, S. Y., Lin, H. H., and Tsauo, J. Y. (2012). Exercise adherence to pelvic floor muscle strengthening is not a significant predictor of symptom reduction for women with urinary incontinence. *Arch. Phys. Med. Rehabil.*, 93(10), 1795-1800.

[232] Burns, P. A., Pranikoff, K., Nochajski, T. H., Hadley, E. C., Levy, K. J., and Ory, M. G. (1993). A comparison of effectiveness of biofeedback and pelvic muscle exercise treatment of stress incontinence in older community-dwelling women. *J. Gerontol.*, 48, 167-174.

[233] Theofrastous, J. P., Wyman, J. F., Bump, R. C., et al. (2002). Effects of pelvic floor muscle training on strength and predictors of response in the treatment of urinary incontinence. *Neurourol. Urodyn.*, 21(5), 486-490.

[234] Bø, K., A H Haakstad, L. and Voldner, N. (2007). Do pregnant women exercise their pelvic floor muscles? *Int. Urogynecol. J. Pelvic Floor Dysfunct.*, 18(7), 733-736.

[235] Jette, A. M. (1982). Improving patient cooperation with arthritis treatment regimens. *Arthritis Rheum.*, 25, 447-453.

[236] Mason, L., Glenn, S., Walton, I., and Hughes, C. (2001). Women's reluctance to seek help for stress incontinence during pregnancy and following childbirth. *Midwifery*, 17(3), 212-221.

[237] McLennan, M. T., Melick, C. F., Alten, B., Young, J., and Hoehn, M. R. (2006). Patients' knowledge of potential pelvic floor changes associated with pregnancy and delivery. *Int. Urogynecol. J. Pelvic Floor Dysfunct.*, 17(1), 22-26.

[238] Bø, K., Larsen, S., Oseid, S., Kvarstein, B., Hagen, R., and Jørgensen, J. (1988). Knowledge about and ability to correct pelvic floor muscle exercises in women with urinary stress incontinence. *Neurourol. Urodyn.*, 7, 261-262.

[239] Holley, R. L., Varner, R. E., Kerns, D. J., and Mestecky, P. J. (1995). Long-term failure of pelvic floor musculature exercises in treatment of genuine stress incon-tinence. *South Med. J.*, 88, 547-549.

[240] Wilson, P. D., Sammarrai, T. A., Deakin, M., Kolbe, E., and Brown, A. D. (1987). An objective assessment of physiotherapy for female genuine stress incontinence. *Br. J. Obstet. Gynecol.*, 94(6), 575-582.

[241] Hay-Smith, J., Mørkved, S., Fairbrother, K. A., and Herbison, G. P. (2008). Pelvic floor muscle training for prevention and treatment of urinary and faecal incontinence in antenatal and postnatal women. *Cochrane Database Syst. Rev.*, 4, CD007471.

[242] Mørkved, S. and Bø, K. (1997). The effect of postpartum pelvic floor muscle exercise in the prevention and treatment of urinary incontinence. *Int. Urogynecol. J.*, 8, 217-222.

[243] Chiarelli, P. and Cockburn, J. (2002). Promoting urinary continence in woman after delivery: randomized controlled trial. *BMJ*, 324, 1241-1246.

[244] Sangi-Haghpeykar, H., Mozayeni, P., Young, A., and Fine, P. M. (2008). Stress urinary incontinence and counseling and practice of pelvic floor exercises postpartum in low-income Hispanic women. *Int. Urogynecol. J. Pelvic Floor Dysfunct.*, 19(3), 361-365.

[245] Chiarelli, P., Murphy, B. and Cockburn, J. (2003). Acceptability of a urinary continence promotion programme to women in postpartum. *Br. J. Obstet. Gynecol.*, 110(2),188-196.

[246] Joanna Briggs Institute. (2006). A pelvic floor muscle exercise programme for urinary incontinence following childbirth. *Nurs. Stand.*, 20(33), 46-50.

[247] Goldstein, M., Hawthorne, M. E., Engeberg, S., McDowell, B. J., and Burgio, K. L. (1992). Urinary incontinence. Why people do not seek help. *J. Gerontol. Nurs.*, 18(4), 15-20.

[248] Peeker, I. and Peeker, R. (2003). Early diagnosis and treatment of genuine stress urinary incontinence in women after pregnancy: midwives as detectives. *J. Midwifery Womens Health*, 48(1), 60-66.

[249] Jain, P. and Parsons, M. (2011). The effects of obesity on the pelvic floor. *The Obstetrician and Gynaecologist*, 13, 133-142.

[250] Subak, L. L., Whitcomb, E., Shen, H., Saxton, J., Vittinghoff, E., and Brown, J. S. (2005). Weight loss: a novel and effective treatment for urinary incontinence. *J. Urol.*, 174, 190-195.

[251] Auwad, W., Steggles, P., Bombieri, L., Waterfield, M., Wilkin, T., and Freeman, R. (2008). Moderate weight loss in obese women with urinary incontinence: a prospective longitudinal study. *Int. Urogynecol. J. Pelvic Floor Dysfunct.*, 19, 1251-1259.

[252] Rasmussen, K. M. and Yaktine, A. L., (2009). *Weight gain during pregnancy: reexamining the guidelines.* Washington DC, National: Academy Press.

[253] Brink, C. A., Sampselle, C. M., Wells, T. J., Diokno, A. C., and Gillis, G. L. (1989). A digital test for pelvic muscle strength in older women with urinary incontinence. *Nurs. Res.*, 38(4), 196-199.

INDEX

A

B

C

D

I

J

K

L

O

P

Q

R

S

Y